90 DAYS to a NEW YOU

The Angela Jordan System

Angela Jordan, M.Y.P., C.F.T

CAJAC Corp.

CAJAC Corp.
10645 N. Tatum Blvd. Suite 200-447
Phoenix, AZ 85028

LCCN 2009906754
ISBN-10 0-615-29726-9
ISBN-13 978-0-615-29726-2
Copyright information available upon request.

Cover Design: Julie Tanner of Brand Canyon Co.
Interior Design: J. L. Saloff
Typography: Adobe Garamond Pro, Myriad Pro,
Bernard MT Condensed, Arial Narrow

v.. 1.0
First Edition, 2009
Printed on acid-free paper.

"Those who say it can't be done should stay out of the way of those already doing it."
— *Unknown*

Rose Lanier: The Detox works! Once I wrapped my mind around preparing my meals ahead of time, the weight just fell off! Low calorie/low carb diets are a thing of my past! The Detox has kicked my metabolism into high gear, allowing me to keep my amazing body, while still enjoying my favorite foods.

✳

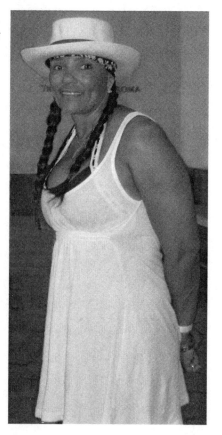

ROSE WORKED OUT WITH ME TWICE A WEEK FOR only 30 minutes each. She tried The Detox a couple of times but would stop after a week because her meals weren't prepared ahead of time. At age 53, Rose has four kids and is definitely an inspiration not only to her family but to all who meet her.

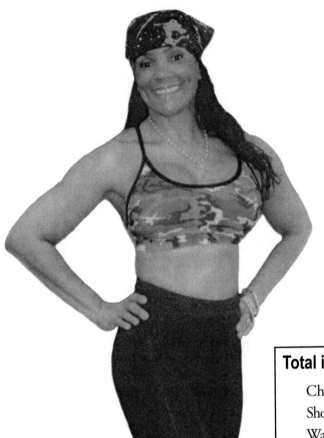

Total inches lost: 27 inches!

Chest- 4	Thigh- 4
Shoulders- 3	Calf- 2
Waist- 6	Bicep- 3
Hips- 5	

Rose Lanier, age 53,
after using the Angela Jordan System
for 90 days.

www.NinetyDaysToANewYou.com

TABLE OF CONTENTS

PART I: 90 Days to a New You
Nutrition Made Simple
Removing Emotional Blocks
Learning About Food and Cooking

Recipes

PART II: 90 Days to a New You
Exercises With Illustrations

Exercises

PART III: 90 Days to a New You
The Detox Program

NOTICE !

Please Read First!

All information contained in this book is intended to supplement and not necessarily replace your present exercise training. It must be understood that all forms of exercise pose some inherent risks. The author and publisher advise all readers to take full responsibility for their own safety and know their own personal limits. Do not take risks beyond your personal level of experience, aptitude, training, and fitness. You must not substitute this exercise routine or dietary regimen for present programs that have been prescribed by your doctor. As with any exercise and/or dietary program, you must get your doctor's approval prior to beginning.

INTRODUCTION

Why Should You Listen to Me?

WITH 32 YEARS OF ENGAGING IN FITNESS AND HEALTH, I HAVE DEVELOPED THE ANGELA Jordan System. Through hard-earned, hands-on education, I have developed a system to help you understand nutrition, learn how to workout effectively, lose weight in a healthy manner, and give you the knowledge to keep it off.

Before I get carried away with talking about The Angela Jordan System, I would like to tell you a little bit about myself. Being athletically gifted and having a "no fear" attitude, I started gymnastics at age five. For the next 11 years, I trained, competed, and learned how to "eat like a winner." I learned the importance of nutrition accompanied by physical conditioning to help my body perform at its best.

Becoming too tall for gymnastics, I went into cheerleading and modeling for two years. I learned how to manipulate my food intake for appearance purposes. Anorexia was rampant.

At 18, I started bodybuilding and began my education in gym management by assisting an owner in running his new gym in Illinois. I learned that muscle mass weighs more than body fat. I learned how to eat for improved muscle function and recovery and also for a lean physical appearance. I did this while recovering from anorexia and

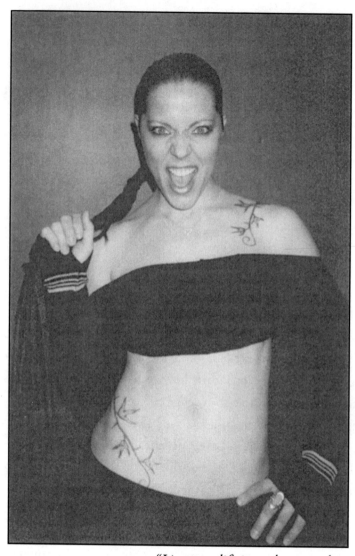

*"Live your life in such a way that
when your feet hit the floor in the morning,
the world shudders and says "Oh hell.....She's awake!"
—Unknown*

by prioritizing nutrition again. I won the title of Ms. Copper Classic Arizona.

Wanting to use my gymnastic abilities, I switched from bodybuilding to fitness competitions. I learned how to really dial in my nutrition and maximize my fitness skills in a new way to perform a two-minute, high-energy, athletically charged fitness routine. I placed in several competitions, including taking 5th in the USAs in Las Vegas, my first national competition. I performed on ESPN and was featured in fitness magazines, including, *Iron Man Magazine, MuscleMag*, and *Joe Weider's 1999 FLEX Magazine Swimsuit Issue*.

I wanted to lose some of my muscle mass so I trained in boxing and kickboxing for two years. My nutrition was focused mostly on muscle strength, stamina, and recovery. I needed strength, speed, and endurance.

While focusing more on my career, I used all of my nutrition and fitness training knowledge and experience to help a professional West Coast hockey team go from last place to winning the cup in a single season. In seven months, I changed their individual body fats from 14% and higher to all of them being under 10%

body fat. With lower body fat, the team skated faster and with sharper technique all the way through the 3rd period while the other team looked like they were skating in sand and were tired. It was a great experience.

Recently, I have been focused on my own gym in Arizona, Camp AJ Athletic Conditioning, and on all my devout clients, helping them stay fit, healthy, and not only have a better quality of life, but also a longer life.

Why Did I Write This Book?

I wanted to wait until I had enough experience, knowledge, and value so people could benefit from my expertise. It's time.

The Angela Jordan System, as defined at the very beginning, has been put to the test, day in and day out, for 32 years in my life and in my gym, and used by hundreds of clients, with proven success. My clients and I have had so much success with my system that they have insisted I put my great information in a book.

I, too, feel it is time to reach as many people in the world as I can with my knowledge. I know my system works, not only because of my clients' successful results, but also because I am living proof.

On a daily basis, my lifestyle and I are the inspiration and motivation that pushes my clients to success and shows them that their goals are attainable. My clients are always amazed that I work 12–14 hour days, starting at 3 a.m., without eating sugar or caffeine, and I am one big ball of energy!

I am about 5'8" and 150 pounds which also baffles my clients. The majority of them guess my weight at least 15 pounds lighter and my age at least 10 years younger. Looking the way I do, at my weight, helps them understand that muscle weighs more than fat and that your weight is just a number. Because of eating so healthy, my skin is very healthy and has a youthful glow. Once I tell them my age, they ask me for my nutrition program because they think it's the fountain of youth.

What's in This Book That's So Good for You?

In PART I, I cover everything from the basics of nutrition to meal plans and recipes, tips on losing weight, ideas to help your kids practice healthy habits, and ways to remove emotional blocks, which, in turn, will help you understand and control your eating habits in the future.

The basics of nutrition will explain just that, what a protein is and what the different carbs and fats are. I give you this information in simple, easy-to-read laymen's terms that even your kids can understand. The meal plans will give you ideas for meals and how to structure your meals for your day. My recipes are very simple and quick to make. I've also given you many other ideas and tips for losing weight, which can be as simple as chewing your food more thoroughly. For your family, I give you easy, helpful tips on how to create healthy habits for your kids. Since the majority of eating problems involve emotions, I go into several ways to face your emotional eating head-on.

In PART II, I have developed my fitness system which is my Functional Freestyle Fitness workout. Functional means using the body to do the move without relying on a machine. Freestyle means using the upper and lower body at the same time. My program allows you variety by letting you pick your own exercises for your workout. I teach you about quality versus quantity and about using intensity to maximize your results. Your workouts are only 20–30 minutes, max!

In PART III, I describe my nationally famous 90-Day Detox program, which not only helps you lose weight and inches but also teaches you about your body and how it reacts to certain foods. My Detox refers to the process of identifying foods that are toxic or damaging to your body, and removing them from or minimizing them in your diet. Once you have finished the 90 days, you will definitely know your body better than you ever have in your whole life. I have people come into my gym just to get The Detox program. My Detox program has changed lives forever.

===

"I can't believe how much food you have to eat on this program."

===

In this book, I will take you through the 90-Day Detox, step by step. I have also included a few testimonials from some of my clients. One of the most common comments my clients make about the 90-Day Detox is, "I can't believe how much food you have to eat on this program." One of the other comments my clients make is, "No matter what diets I have been on in the past, the 90-Day Detox fits every lifestyle." And my favorite comment is, "The 90-Day Detox literally changed my relationship with food."

What Are You Going to Get From This Book?

It's your lucky day! Through the years, I have listened to all the clients who have come through my gym complain about other nutrition programs and other nutrition books. Some common complaints were: too complex, too hard to understand, a lot of extra nonsense they didn't care to know, and the two biggest complaints: always hungry, and didn't fit my lifestyle.

One of the biggest things I have learned from all of my clients is they don't want to hear all the fancy formulas and clinical vocabulary. They just want to fit into their clothes better, walk up the stairs without being out of breath, and most importantly, they want a better quality of life. They want the information quick, simple, and effective.

Behold! In your hands, *90 Days to a New You*, is just that book! I have given you The Angela Jordan System in laymen's terms, to the point, and with the knowledge on how to apply them to your life today, tomorrow, and always.

Within these pages, you will receive the knowledge to not only change physically from the inside out but also mentally and emotionally. In my chapter, "Get R.E.A.L.," I will take you through the steps that put you face-to-face with your eating habits and the emotions that go with them.

I have had female clients regulate their PMS and stop the hot flashes of menopause.

I have had clients lower their blood pressure, get the lowest cholesterol reading they've ever had in their entire life, and regulate their insulin to stop type 2 diabetes. I have had female clients regulate their PMS and stop the hot flashes of menopause. Clients sleep better than they have ever slept. The Detox has cleared up skin conditions and relieved headaches and joint aches.

Don't even get me started on the inches these clients lose! Three inches off their waist in the first two weeks; 6-8 inches off their waist after the first 30 days. This program works!

Emotionally and mentally, I am with you every step of the way. Through working one-on-one with so many clients, I have learned how to motivate, support, and supply you with the right tools to keep you moving forward. I don't just throw the information at you and say good luck. I will guide you on how to take my information and apply it to your life to make the changes you need to reach your goals.

Once you commit to my program, you will be like all of my successful clients who now say, "The Angela Jordan System has released the athlete within me, and this book will be my primary resource for health and well-being."

90 DAYS
TO A NEW YOU

PART I

Nutrition Made Simple
Removing Emotional Blocks
Learning About Food and Cooking

1 YOU HOLD THE KEY

"When I let go of what I am, I become what I might be."
—Lao Tzu

THERE IS ONLY ONE "YOU" IN THIS WORLD, AND WE NEED YOU. EVERYONE HAS A purpose. Your purpose here is no less then anyone else's purpose. There are many people who count on your presence in their lives and would be very upset if you were no longer here.

You and your health are first priority in your life. If you don't take care of "YOU," there will be no "YOU" to take care of the many people who count on you every day. You are so special and so unique that only "YOU" can fulfill certain needs of others. You are quite a creation and there is no other. There is no "practice life." You only get this life.

You have selected my book for a reason. You are ready to feel better, get healthier, and have a better quality of life. You are ready to take charge of your life, become one with your mind, body, and spirit, and to honor the one and only YOU.

YOU HOLD THE KEY to unlocking your powers to put my information to good use. It's really simple, as you will soon read. There are no secrets, no gimmicks, and no fast, easy ways to do this. You are holding all the answers in your hands right now. You just have to use the information and reap the rewards. No one can lose weight for you.

You have to do this for yourself. I am here to motivate you enough to change your life before your health decides to do it for you.

Believe It
Be It
Become It

Whatever you BELIEVE about yourself you will start to BE or function as that belief which will eventually make you BECOME IT. Think about that for a minute. If you believe you will always be overweight, you will become overweight. If you believe you can't eat right, you will eat badly all the time and you will become an out-of-control bad eater. On the other hand, if you BELIEVE you will always BE fit, you will BECOME fit. If you BELIEVE you can eat right, you will BE a better eater all the time and you will BECOME a healthier eater.

I explain to my clients that when a person wants something and believes they can accomplish it, they will do whatever it takes to become it. For example, a first-time mother wants to be the best mom. She will buy every baby book ever written; she will eat healthy. She will make all the right choices for her firstborn to have every chance to have perfect health.

Another example is the corporate guy who starts at the bottom of the company. He decides he wants to be in the top position so he learns everything possible, works all the extra hours, and goes those extra miles to get there.

Your eating habits are the same. This book will give you the body you want. Your body will feel strong and function strong, just like a professional athlete, making you realize you have now released the athlete within you.

This book will improve your health and change your life forever. This book

> I am here to motivate you enough to change your life before your health decides to do it for you.

will change not only your relationship with your body but also your relationship with food. You will succeed! There is no other way to think. So, if you have a belief of failure in you right now, maybe you're not ready to make the commitment to change. If you are ready to succeed and accomplish that goal you've set for yourself, read on and let me show you the way! To keep you focused, I recommend you ask yourself on a daily basis,

What Do I Believe?
What Am I Being?
What Am I Becoming?

===

It's time you get serious and take control of your body, your health, and your life.

===

NO one can do this for you but I promise to be with you every step of the way. I will teach you not only how to eat but also ways to see why you eat the way you do. I am going to explain different ways to lose weight. It is your choice on how intense you want to take it.

Remember, we are striving for a life-style change not a quick fix. I will help you through all the emotions and physical changes you will go through when you change your eating habits. All you have to do is be honest with yourself and stick with me no matter how many times you want to go back to your old habits. I know you can do this, and you know you can do this.

I'm sure this is not the first nutrition book you have ever bought but I would like it to be the last nutrition book you'll ever need. You can read every nutrition book out there, but until you decide to make the right choices you'll end up right back where you started—lost, depressed, discouraged, and back at square one. I don't want this to be another nutrition book on your shelf.

All you have to remember is that YOU HOLD THE KEY to your health and well-being. I'm just going to give you the answers on how to use your key. Help me to help you, and decide TODAY that you are going to start being responsible for what you are feeding your body.

Stay focused, stay positive, and stay with me through this wonderful learning experience, and this will definitely be the last nutrition book you will ever need.

2 LET'S GET OUR FEET WET

"If you think you can do a thing, or think you can't do a thing, you're right."
–Henry Ford

SOME PEOPLE LIKE TO RUN AND JUMP INTO THE POOL. OTHERS LIKE TO STAND ON THAT first step and just get their feet wet, slowly getting used to that water. If you're in the first group, you've probably tried some extreme measures for losing weight without any hesitation. If you are in the second group, you will probably need a different approach to your weight loss that matches that of getting into a cold pool, slow with some hesitation. I've included every different type of personality in my quest to help you lose weight.

What I am saying is that I have worked one-on-one with clients for almost 20 years and on my own weight, personally and professionally, for 32 years, and I totally understand that you're not all the same physically, mentally, or emotionally. Therefore, I'm not going to treat everyone the same. If you're in the second group, you have probably already bought every diet book out there, having little to no success with your weight loss.

This book is not your normal diet book. Stick with me; I'll get you to your goals. Keep an open mind and try to resist negative thoughts toward my directions and you will accomplish your goals so much faster and with less negativity.

Now, if you're in the first group, where you plunge right into that pool, you're probably someone who has said, "I'll try anything once," without asking too many questions or having too many concerns. If it doesn't work out, no love lost, and no big deal.

of these descriptions. Usually, it will also follow suit with how they run their lives. It's kind of like how different people deal with change.

Some people want to dwell on all the things they no longer have. Others embrace the new and can't even remember

You have to take responsibility for the change of your own health.

The second group, on the other hand, is not as easygoing. No matter how much you splash them or try to coax or cheer them into jumping into that pool, they are resistant to the point where some of them just turn around and step back out of that pool altogether. This group tends to be ruled by their emotions, and is usually very reluctant to change. Unless it's their idea, it's no go. Your persuasiveness actually makes this type of person rebel and do the opposite of what you're trying to help them through.

Gosh, all that from two different people entering a cold pool. But think about it. I guarantee you can name two people you know or have known who fits one

what the old used to be. So how do you want to treat your health? Do you want to step into that cold pool slowly, starting at the top step, looking back at that nice warm towel you just had wrapped around you? Or do you want to take charge of your health, and jump right in wholeheartedly, never looking back! It's up to you, but make sure that your choice fits your needs and is a choice that you can commit to. Pick YOUR approach to assure YOUR success.

No one else can do this for you, which I hope you know by now. As much as I want this for you, it's your health, not mine. You have to want this, not your mate, not your family, not your friends, not your healthcare providers. You have to take responsibility for the change of your own health.

There are people like me who can give you the answers you need, to make the road less rocky, but I can't drive the car for you. It's up to you to apply the information to fit your lifestyle and make it work for you. Only you know what makes you tick.

Even when my clients tell me, "I just love the taste of food," there is a deep-seated reason they eat in abundance or uncontrollably.

A lot of people will say they don't know what makes them tick, but they do know. They're just not ready to take responsibility and face the reasons they've failed in the past.

After 20 years of working with people who try to tell me, "I don't know why I eat the way I do," they all end up eventually crying or getting angry with themselves and finally breaking down and telling me the real reasons. For example, marriage issues, career discontent, and loneliness are just few.

If you can go deep inside yourself, and be true to yourself, to find the real reason or reasons you eat the way you do, write it down, face it head-on, and conquer it! Later, I will give you a chance to journal your thoughts and progress, which will keep you true to yourself and your actions. All my clients journal and keep a food log that I check once a week to keep them honest with themselves and with me. I highly recommend that everyone have a supportive person who will keep you honest by reviewing your journal with you. Once you can successfully do this, your food issues will go away.

Even when my clients tell me, "I just love the taste of food," there is a deep seated reason they eat in abundance or uncontrollably. There is a reason they are always pulled toward certain "comfort foods." So let's get to your core reason so you can stop calling food the enemy.

Use the following pages to write your thoughts on how you deal with change, and how you feel about your personal goals and accomplishing them.

_____

_____

_____

_____

_____

_____

_____

_____

_____

_____

_____

_____

_____

_____

_____

_____

_____

_____

_____

_____

_____

_____

_____

_____

_____

_____

_____

_____

_____

_____

_____

_____

_____

_____

_____

3 EMOTIONS RUN WILD

"Be miserable. Or motivate yourself. Whatever has to be done, it's always your choice."
—Wayne Dyer

"I feel: unloved, unattractive, lonely, sad, angry, bored, unhappy, lost, rejected, stressed, anxious, depressed, tired, abused, comforted, rewarded, bitter, like celebrating, like a failure, in denial, like escaping, etc."

EMOTIONAL EATING IS ONE OF THE MAIN CAUSES FOR GAINING WEIGHT. I GUARANTEE you have eaten for one or more of the reasons above. Everyone does it at some point or another. I did. It's when it becomes a habit that it becomes harmful to your body.

When it comes to your eating habits, you have to be honest with yourself. People always ask me, "What diet works?" My answer, "The one you stick to." The saying, "You are what you eat," is so true. The next time you're at a restaurant or a supermarket, check out what other people are eating or buying and then see if it matches the physical health/appearance of that person. The majority of the time, it will.

No matter what nutrition program you follow, healthy or unhealthy, your body tells the truth. Until you get real and take a good look as to the reasons you eat the way you do, you'll never be able to control your weight. Therefore, you keep running into the same problems over and over.

A good way to see your emotional reasons for eating is by trying a new, healthy eating program. What will happen is you will crave your comfort foods, which you cannot have, nor does your body need. Your mind wants it.

A well-balanced nutrition program has all the nutrients it needs, plus plenty of food. So, when you are freaking out and stressing about a piece of chocolate or a soda, and you really can't make it through the day without this one little treat, you really need to ask yourself, what am I not emotionally dealing with,

I had a client tell me she was on the verge of buying the next size up in jeans, and she really didn't want to have to do that. She asked me what she could change in her eating habits that would help her drop a couple of pounds without going too extreme. I asked her to give me an example of a typical day or a couple of days of what she eats. I needed to know not only what she ate, but also how much and at what times.

She had a 32-oz Pepsi™ every day, and ate around 8–10 Hershey Kisses™ throughout the day. She ate a small salad

What are you willing to do and what are you willing to settle for, when it comes to the shape of your body.

or what's missing in my life that I can't be without this little piece of food. You may just say, "Because I want it, and I don't deprive myself." That's great! Now you know why you eat the way you do and why your weight is where it is. So, enjoy your food and enjoy your shape. I mean seriously, you can't have it all!

for lunch with no complex carbs or protein. She ate out for dinner, usually a large meal, like pasta. I told her to start eating breakfast, drop the Pepsi™, and cut the amount of chocolate in half. I told her to eat the pasta at lunch and eat the salad at dinner, adding protein to it.

She didn't want to drop the Pepsi™

cold turkey. I told her she could have two chocolates and one can of Pepsi™, but not the 32-oz. size. She told me she hated breakfast, wanted three cans of Pepsi™ and couldn't promise me what she could eat at dinner because her husband picked the restaurant. By the end of our half-hour training session, it was clear to me my client was not ready to really change anything.

When a person really wants something, they will commit, make the changes, and do whatever it takes to make that goal.

So guess what I said to her? "Enjoy drinking your 32-oz. Pepsi™, as you drive to the mall to buy the next size up in jeans. You don't want this bad enough." She looked at me so confused. I told her if the next size up really bothered her, she would do whatever it takes to avoid having to go up a jean size.

I wasn't even making it that strict for her and she still chose to rebel and refused to change her wants.

I told her, as I have written earlier, when a woman becomes pregnant for the first time, she reads everything she can get her hands on to be the best mother. Just like the new office worker doing all the hours and extra work to climb that corporate ladder to get the top position in the company. When a person really wants something, they will commit, make the changes, and do whatever it takes to make that goal. They have a will inside them and a focus that is unstoppable!

This is what I explain during every nutrition consultation I go through. What you want has to be more than what you already have. After 20 years of working one-on-one with people, I can tell who's serious and ready, and who is not. So, when it comes to your eating habits, you have to ask yourself, how bad do you want it?

Another good story along these lines began with me standing in line at Costco. I was buying my three cases of canned tuna in water, not oil, when a woman came up behind me and said, "I bet you don't put mayonnaise on that." I said, "No, I eat it right out of the can." She said, "That's what I thought. Well, you can have your cute little butt. That is not worth it to me."

So there is another question you must ask yourself when it comes to your eating habits and the shape of your body. What are you willing to do and what are you willing to settle for when it comes to the shape of your body?

Emotional baggage can be so strong. You can't even believe how much it is controlling you. Some eating habits have been programmed in as early as when you were a kid. My dad was raised in a house with two brothers. All three boys were athletic and big eaters. His parents didn't have a lot of money and his dad worked in a bakery. His dad was able to take home any of the day-old bread that was expired by one day, for free.

His mother took advantage of this by making big pots of bean soups, which lasted for days. She poured it over four pieces of toast for her boys. For breakfast, she poured milk and sugar over four pieces of toast. The boys ate a lot of peanut butter and jelly sandwiches. She used bread to fill them up because they couldn't afford a lot of expensive meals.

When I asked my dad to share his eating habits from when he was a kid, he had a huge "light bulb moment" right in front of me! At his current age of 56 years old, he finally realized why he struggles with eating a lot of breads, muffins, pan-cakes, etc. He said even if he had a nice steak dinner with veggies and a baked potato, he was never satisfied unless he had bread with his meal.

Emotional blocks affect everyone, from men to women, young to old, athletic or not.

He suddenly realized he mentally does not feel full unless he has bread. He also realized that when he's emotional in any way, stressed, happy, or sad, bread makes everything better. Now that he found his reason for his eating habits, he had to change it. I put him on The Angela Jordan System, which he followed to a T. I then put him on a maintenance program, which he still follows today. I am happy to report that not only has he lost over 75 pounds, he still enjoys bread, but in moderation, and not as his main course of the meal.

Emotional blocks affect everyone, from men to women, young to old, athletic or not. I've worked with men and women of all ages, from eight years old to 87 years old. I've worked with clients with many different needs, circumstances, and emotional blocks. I've worked with a teenage boy needing to add more strength and size for football, a 42-year-old housewife with two kids who wanted her fit body back, a paraplegic who needed to strengthen his upper body to make his transfers easier, a 50-year-old diabetic who needed to get her weight down and her blood sugar under control, and finally, a professional athlete who needed to be leaner and improve his speed skills to improve his game. There is one thing they all have in common. They are all human.

What I mean is, they all have the same basic ingredients inside them and they all have emotions. Each person wants to focus on certain parts of their body, but they still have to follow some basic rules to achieve their goals.

There are no quick fixes. There are no magic pills. There are no easy remedies. You have to start taking responsibility for what you are feeding your body. Eating is purely for survival, so your body does not starve to death. It's our emotions that say, "I need to eat this whole container of ice cream."

Consciously, you know how to eat. You know what's right and what's wrong. It's the issues that lie subconsciously or even consciously that lead you down the wrong path.

No matter who you are, until you understand why you eat the way you do, you will continue to struggle with your weight issues. With my book and your motivation you will understand and control your emotional eating forever.

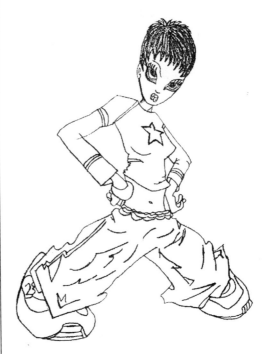

**"Control emotional eating...
change your eating habits
FOREVER!"**

On the following pages, write your thoughts on your emotional attachments to food. Do you overeat or deprive yourself, and what satisfaction do you get from this act.

4 HOW THE MACHINE (YOUR BODY) RUNS

"No matter how hard you beat yourself up in the gym, if you do not change the stuff going on inside, the outside will not respond as expected."

WORKING WITH MY MANY CLIENTS THROUGH THE YEARS, I HAVE FOUND THAT FOOD IS the main reason a body will or will not change. No matter how hard you beat yourself up in the gym, if you do not change the stuff going on inside, the outside will not respond as expected.

When I am talking about function, not appearance, I like to use the comparison of your car and your body. If your car, which is a machine, does not have the right stuff on the inside, it will not function at its best—just like your body. I am going completely on function with this and how people don't understand why they feel so bad or why they can't function as well as they used to.

Your car is a predictable machine that responds, good or bad, depending on the type of fuel and care that is given to its working parts. Your body responds with the same predictability. I know people who treat their car better than they treat their body. Imagine if you never changed the oil or put the wrong kind of gas in your car. Over time, how well would your car run? Now how about when you go to the gym every day

31

and beat yourself up for hours then you don't put the right foods in to your body to make it function at its best?

If you never change the oil in your car and forget to put gas in the tank, you're not going to get very far. Your body is like your car, it should be a fine-tuned machine. I've watched clients not eat certain foods their body needs then wonder why they feel like they do. I've watched clients go all day without taking the time like to combine different ways of eating to keep the body from getting into a rut. You definitely need a cheat day or maybe some of you even need a little cheat every day. Not only does this keep the mind stable, but it also challenges the body every day with something different.

A key to keeping your weight under control is to keep your metabolism going strong by feeding it. It is important to understand that metabolic rates, as a rule,

People who say they can go all day not eating, without ever feeling hungry, shouldn't be proud of that.

to eat and then wonder why they can't function very well.

Now let's go back to that beautiful car of yours. Stop putting in some of the fluids it needs to run and see how long your fine-tuned machine lasts you. I'm going to give you the basics on what your fine-tuned machine, your body, needs to function at its best.

I will educate you about food and how to keep eating and feeding yourself in the right ways. I believe in moderation and I are created not inherited. Everyone has that friend or relative who is always eating ever time you see them, yet they stay thin. The reason is, they are constantly putting in fuel for the body to use, so there is no reason to store extra body fat for survival purposes.

Every meal you skip, your body will hold on to more of the next one, storing it into your fat cells for later. What?! Yes, you heard me right. For every meal you skip your body stores more of the next meal in your fat cells. Why?! Your body doesn't understand when you are going to eat or skip another meal, so it makes sure to get enough out of this meal to keep you functioning. If you can get on a regular schedule of eating throughout your day, the body has no reason to store so much. Your body knows it will get another meal soon, so it starts burning the current meal for energy.

People who say they can go all day without eating, and they don't even feel hungry, shouldn't be proud of that. Their metabolism has pretty much shut down. Not only are they not burning fat, because the body is totally storing it so they don't pass out, but they are also losing muscle.

You have to keep fueling the body to keep that fat-burning process going.

The body will eat away at muscle to use for energy and strength to get them through their long day. Imagine a little fire burning in our stomach, melting that body fat away. The only way to keep a fire going is to feed it with wood, right? You have to keep fueling the body to keep that fat-burning process going. Feed that fire! Keep that baby burning!

One way you can tell if your metabolism has slowed is if your extremities, your arms and legs, but mainly your hands and feet, are always cold, even if it's warm outside. Your body holds the heat in your middle to protect your organs.

A more scientific way to see if your metabolism is working and you are burning fat, is to take your temperature in the morning. I did this when I competed in fitness competitions. Before you start a new nutrition program, take your morning temperature every morning for one week. Keep the thermometer next to the bed. When you awake, try not to move much by reaching over to grab the thermometer. Record each day, and find your average temperature at the end of the week. This will be your normal temperature. This number may be different from everyone else's; remember, it's YOUR temperature.

Once you start a new nutrition program, take your morning temperature and record it every day or even once or twice a week. If you notice the temperature is dropping, it means your metabolism is getting slower, not faster. This means you're probably not burning fat. Once in awhile your temperature will drop, but if it stays low or continues to drop quite often, you will need to change your nutrition program. More than likely you will need to up your food intake with more healthy, nutritious foods, and your temperature will go up, which will indicate that you are burning more fat. Remember, eat right, eat more, burn more

---

A key to keeping your weight under control is to keep your metabolism going strong by feeding it.

The average human body burns up most of a meal in three hours and is ready to take on the next meal for more fuel. Think about it. You eat breakfast before you go to work around 7 a.m. Around 10 a.m. you are hungry but feel you should hold out until lunch. Wrong! This same thing usually happens after lunch, which is around noon or 1 p.m. At around 3:30–4 p.m., you start feeling hungry but feel you should hold out until dinner at six. Wrong again! You should have breakfast, lunch, dinner, and two more meals, one midmorning, and one midafternoon.

Now that is not set in stone for every day. I'm not telling you that you have to eat five meals every day. I'm also not going to tell you when to start or when to stop eating those meals. I don't know your schedule. I have a hard enough time keeping up with my own. I'm just telling you how the human body works. It's up to you to look at your lifestyle and your schedule, and make it fit you.

I, for example, work 14 hours on many days. I am up at 2:45 a.m. and in bed by around 9 or 10 p.m. I know, I know, not enough sleep. I am working on that. I doubt many of you are eating your breakfast at 4 a.m., but I would like to illustrate that you can make this work. Your first meal needs to start an hour after you awake. I am extremely active running my gym, training 25–30 people a day. I'm throwing medicine balls, lifting weights for the clients, and holding the mitts for my boxing clients. My body likes to get fuel every 2 ½-3 hours. My first meal is around 4 a.m. and my last meal is around 6:30–7:30, depending on when I can get to bed.

You want to eat your last meal three hours before bed. Not one, not two, I said three. Not only for the purpose of burning that meal with movement before going to sleep, but also so your stomach, the actual organ, is not full. When you sleep, your stomach muscles relax. If your stomach is full, it will push your belly out, eventually giving you a distended gut in your lower abdominal area, and you won't have the benefit of movement to burn the food your stomach is filled with.

Your nutrition program has to fit your lifestyle.

Now what I meant earlier about the number of meals per day not being set in stone is that your lifestyle is not the same every day. I, for example, am a workaholic for six days a week until Sunday arrives. Instead of getting out of bed at 2:45 a.m., like I do during the week, I'm lucky if I get out of bed before noon. I try not to do too much physical activity, maybe catch a movie, read books, and I tend to go to bed earlier, like around 7 p.m.

So you can see that during my work week I may average six or seven meals a day. On Sundays, I may only get 2-3 meals in, because I'm sleeping the rest of the time. I call my Sundays "recharge-my-battery day." So do you understand what I'm saying when I say, "Your nutrition program has to fit your lifestyle." A third-shift worker would have a different eating schedule than a first-shift worker. Understand? I also tell people, "Eat for what you are about to do." Translation— you don't need a huge meal to go sit on the couch and watch TV. Adjust what you eat for your planned activity.

Once you awake, the size of your meals through your day should follow the shape of a triangle.

Your breakfast should be your biggest meal of the day. Your midmorning meal should be a bit smaller, but not by much. Your lunch is your last hurrah, and your midafternoon meal and dinner should be smaller. Your dinner is the smallest meal of the day. You are eating for the bulk of the activity of your day. Whether you are a first- or a third-shift person, your meals should follow the triangle. At the end of your workday, you wind down. You watch TV, sit at the computer, read, and relax.

I find that most of you have an upside-down triangle. You eat little to no breakfast, a bit bigger lunch, and a huge dinner! There is another group of people that eat like the shape of the hourglass. They get a good breakfast but then skip meals all day, only to make up for it with a huge dinner. Most of the reasons for eating the wrong way are: no time, slept in, no food readily available. So which way do you eat, the triangle, the upside-down triangle, or the hourglass? What are your reasons?

So, now you know:

Eat a meal every three hours, starting with your first meal and an hour after you awake.

Allow three hours after your last meal to properly digest your meal before you go to bed.

Eat for your upcoming activity level; eat for what you're going to do.

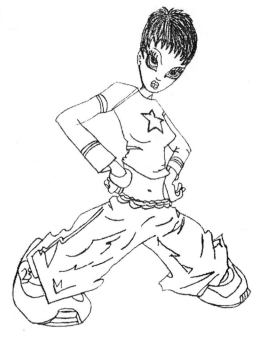

"Respect your body... you only have one!"

5 WHAT'S IN A COMPLETE MEAL? PROTEINS

WHEN YOU SIT DOWN TO EAT, YOU WANT A COMPLETE MEAL. NOT A SNACK, LIKE A handful of nuts. Your body does a lot for you. I think it deserves more than a handful of nuts. The first thing you need to see in your meal is protein.

Now I'm going to keep my promise and not get all technical on you. This is how I've explained nutrition to my clients for 20 years. They have all been relieved to finally know what a protein does. So here we go.

Protein: feeds the muscles, helps them recover, helps with strength and hardness, and helps create size. Protein helps with hair and nail strength and growth. It helps stabilize blood sugar and slows down carbohydrate absorption.

There are two types of proteins, complete and incomplete. Complete proteins contain the proper amount of amino acids that your body requires. An incomplete protein does not. Amino acids are the building blocks of protein. They are a major source of energy for your body and are produced by your own body. They help us maintain muscle tone and are depleted by physical activity and other stresses on the body. The only way to replenish your amino acids is to eat complete proteins. So what are some examples of a complete protein?

Complete Proteins: beef, chicken, turkey, fish, eggs, and soy

As you will notice, a complete protein comes from an animal source which also produces its own amino acids. The exception to this rule is soy, which is the only known complete protein derived from a plant source.

By now you have probably guessed, an incomplete protein does not come from an animal and when eaten alone does not have a sufficient amount of amino acids required for your body. Some examples of incomplete proteins follow:

**peanut butter,
some protein drinks,
cheese,
nuts, quinoa,
legumes,
and seeds**

Good plant sources, such as legumes and nuts, combined with whole-grain cereals is an example of combining proteins to form a complete protein to fill your amino acid needs.

If you choose to follow any type of vegetarian diet, consult a nutritionist who is trained in working with this diet. If you do not do a vegetarian diet the right way, your body will be affected from not getting certain nutrients that it needs.

If you are a meat eater, choose a small filet or flank steak, pork chops, pork roast, buffalo burgers, ostrich burgers, and even lamb.

Turkey is easier to digest than chicken because of the connective tissue in chicken. If you boil the chicken, that gets rid of all the connective tissue and makes it very tender.

Fish is one of the leanest proteins, especially cod. Salmon and orange roughy are great sources of protein.

Eggs are the easiest, quickest, most readily digestible protein there is. If your protein intake is too low, a good indication may be some of these side effects: fatigue, lack of muscle recovery, constant burning in the muscles when starting a physical activity, muscle weakness, muscle appearance is flat without hardness or not having a "toned" look, and, finally, you constantly crave sugar. I bet that last one woke you up. Another tidbit that might shock you is, overconsumption of protein can result in excess protein converting to fat. A good rule of thumb is, a portion of protein should be no larger than the palm of your hand, per meal.

6 WHAT'S IN A COMPLETE MEAL? CARBOHYDRATES

THE NEXT THING YOU NEED TO INCLUDE IN YOUR COMPLETE MEAL IS carbohydrates, or carbs, as we all call them. These poor guys have gotten such a bad rap in the past couple of years. To this day, I have clients who are afraid to put them into their mouths when they think of the word "diet." Or they say they are eating plenty of carbs and they name fruits and veggies. I have to tell them they are not eating the right carbs to lose fat. That's when they look at me with that disgusted look, like, "I give up!"

I'll try to make this as simple and painless as possible. Here we go. There are two types of carbs, simple and complex. You want to limit your simple carb intake. Unfortunately, these are the carbs that every one of you enjoys. These are the processed carbs, like: muffins, bagels, cookies, crackers, breads, pastas, cold cereals, and basically anything man-made. Are you depressed yet?

Complex carbs come in two categories, starchy and fibrous. These are the carbs you want to eat in every meal. They help give your body energy so it doesn't need to store fat for energy. Starchy carbs consist of: oatmeal, rice, yams, sweet potatoes, white or red potatoes, cream of rice, cream of wheat, and grits. Fibrous carbs consist of all fruit and veggies. These carbs I call "the bottle brush" for the body. They supply the "roughage" to make you go number two and help clean out your body.

I have added the right carbs to a client's nutrition program, taken away some cardio they were going crazy on, and watched their body get leaner in a matter of two weeks. If you don't get the right amount of the right carbs in the body, it doesn't matter how much cardio you do. Your body will not drop body fat. It may even lose muscle tone, instead.

Carbohydrates stabilize blood sugar, allow the body to burn fat, act as fuel for the body to function, and give the muscles glycogen, which is a technical word for "muscle fuel." Did you know that fat has more than twice the calories of starch, as in carbs. Starchy foods are not fattening, the sauces, butters, jellies, and gravy we put all over them is.

The body actually prefers to convert to body fat the calories from fat over the calories from carbohydrates. If you have two people eat the same amount of calories, one eating the calories in fat and the other in carbohydrates, the person eating the fat will have a tendency to gain more body fat than the other. So eat the carbs with fewer condiments all over them, and in normal portion sizes. Stop being afraid of them!

Good Carbs / Starchy: oatmeal, rice, yams, sweet potatoes, white or red pota-toes, cream of rice, cream of wheat, and grits. These break down slowly in the body and sustain you longer from being hungry or having a low blood sugar moment.

Good Carbs / Fibrous: green veggies, most other veggies, and fruits.

Bad Carbs: muffins, crackers, cookies, cakes, pasta, breads, these are what you limit in your nutrition program because they break down quickly and need to be used as energy.

You need both starchy and fibrous carbs in each meal, except the last meal before bed. You do not need a starchy carb before bed because you are usually sitting around being less active. Your last meal should consist of a protein and some veggies.

Lack of carbs: low in energy, headaches, dizziness, nausea, moodiness, constant cravings for breads, pastas, and sweets.

Let me talk a little bit about insulin and glycogen. I know I said I wouldn't go technical on you, but these are pretty easy to learn. Most people understand insulin is needed to maintain metabolism and stabilize your blood sugar. If your insulin is too low, you are feeling some of the symptoms above. If your insulin is too high, your blood sugar will also be high. This could result in symptoms such as having a headache, being very hyper, feeling sick to your stomach, and then needing a nap when it finally stabilizes. You also tend to have weight gain if you're not secreting enough insulin and your blood sugar is too low.

Glycogen, needed for strength and power, is the storage form of blood sugar in the muscle. It takes your muscles anywhere from 48–72 hours to replenish glycogen levels after a physical activity. You will know your glycogen is too low in your muscles if they are burning and fatigued within the first few minutes of a physical activity. The only way to replenish this glycogen is to eat starchy carbs.

Now here's where it can get a little tricky. Stick with me here. Simple carbs have a very quick absorption in the body. That's why they are called simple. Complex carbs break down slower and sustain your energy level for anywhere

from 2-3 hours after you eat them.

If your blood sugar is low because you just did a huge workout, you replenish the glycogen fast with a simple carb. I understand that I have told you to limit your simple carbs, but they do have a place in your diet because they will replenish your glycogen fast and stabilize your blood sugar almost instantly.

You have a complex carb a couple of hours before the workout to have the right amount of glycogen for your muscles to perform. An example of this would be a chicken-rice bowl with veggies a couple of hours before the workout, and a muffin or even a banana after the workout for immediate sugar replenishing.

Even though fruit is a fibrous, good carb, it is still sugar. I know it's natural, but it's still sugar. Eat the simple carb in the car on the way home from the gym. Once you're home, within the next hour, eat a "complete meal." If you ever have a very low drop in your blood sugar while being active, take a very high sugar substance, immediately.

For instance, I push my clients hard for my famous 30-minute workouts. Sometimes, they suddenly turn white, including their lips, and feel clammy, dizzy, and nauseated. I give them a Jolly Rancher™ hard candy, and within seconds their color comes back and they feel better. I tell them they have to eat a "complete meal" within the next 30 minutes or their blood sugar will drop again. So I suggest that if you know you are going to be very active, you should carry some

because of the insulin surge it gives you if you eat it by itself. If you smear some peanut butter on it, you now change the glycemic load on the body and stabilize your insulin. I suggest that you keep your glycemic load low, unless you need a high glycemic index food immediately after vigorous activity.

For long term, successful weight loss, you must keep complex carbs in your nutrition program.

Jolly Rancher hard candies, to be safe.

I would say the majority of clients I have worked with do not eat enough of the right carbs. This affects not only their workouts, but mainly their weight loss.

There is also glycemic index and glycemic load. Glycemic index is the chart that gives each food an individual number according to the effect it has on the body if it is eaten by itself. These charts are available from your doctor or any health food store. The glycemic load is what you get once you put that food with something else. For example, a rice cake is like eating air. It is high on the glycemic index

Well I hope I haven't confused you. Are you still with me? Great! I knew you could hang with me! You must keep complex carbs in your nutrition program to lose fat. Programs that have you eat high protein and fibrous carbs (vegetables), with no complex carbs, are only tricking you into thinking you've lost body fat.

Complex carbs provide the body with glycogen, which is also stored with water. Therefore, when you take away the complex carbs, your glycogen will get used up, which means you will also lose that extra water you're holding.

The results you get: loss of 10 pounds

in a week! The bad news: gain of 10 pounds and then some within a few days of eating those complex carbs again.

Since these programs are also very low in calories, your body will tend to clean itself out by eliminating any extra waste you've been carrying. Translation, you have some really good poops, which flattens your tummy. Again, this weight loss you will see on the scale is not body fat weight loss.

So, repeat after me. No complex carbs and a low-calorie nutrition program equals: water and waste loss with very little to no body fat loss. Now don't get me wrong. You will feel less bloated and thinner, but it will only be temporary. I will only recommend the no-carb route to clients who have a party or unexpected event they need to attend within the next 1-2 weeks. I just warn them that it will all come back once the event is over and they start eating those carbs again.

If you notice, most programs recommend the no-carb route for the first two weeks. This will do that neat little trick of making you lose water and waste material, making you drop pounds on your scale. They do this because it gives you hope and faith in their program.

Once my clients go into that third or fourth week of those other programs, when they tell you to add oatmeal or a little rice or even fruit, my clients tell me they always gain back a couple of pounds. For long-term, successful weight loss, you must keep complex carbs in your nutrition program.

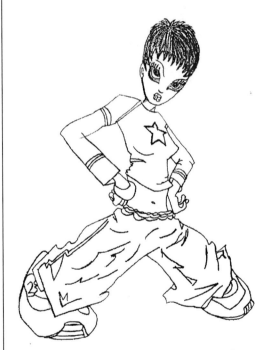

"You need to eat complex carbs to burn fat"

7 WHAT'S IN A COMPLETE MEAL? FATS, GOOD & BAD CHOLESTEROL

NOW LET'S TALK ABOUT THE LAST THING YOU NEED TO HAVE A "COMPLETE MEAL." FAT. Most of you know what the good fats are and what the bad fats are. Maybe not. I'm sure you have all heard of "trans fats." Those are the bad, processed fats you do not want to consume. Many fried and deep-fried foods are cooked in unhealthy, saturated fats (animal fats, lard). Most of the packaging in our supermarkets is now labeled with "no trans fats." For example, peanut butter labels now tell you whether they contain trans fats. Here are the different fats and some examples of each one.

Saturated (bad): processed animal products (hot dogs, lunch meats), high fat dairy products (cheddar cheese, buttermilk), fatty meats, and foods cooked in animal fats.

Saturated (good): lean meats (fish, chicken), low-fat dairy (skim milk, yogurt).

Polyunsaturated (good): corn, soybean, safflower, and sunflower oils.

Monounsaturated (good): vegetable and nut oils, such as olive, peanut, and canola.

It is important to understand that you should include some of each of these categories of fat in your diet. The key is to focus on the better fats and not drown your good, natural foods in unnecessary fats. An example would be to broil your lean steak rather than frying it, bake your chicken rather than fry or deep fry it, and poach or broil your fish rather than fry or deep fry it.

Did you know that if you don't eat enough of the good fats, it could elevate your cholesterol!

When it comes to saturated fats, limit red fatty meats, which do not digest as well. Instead, substitute meats that contain fats that digest easier. An example would be fish, which is a great source of omega fats. These fats, although classified as saturated fats, are easily digested and utilized by the body. I try to eat salmon, which is very high in omega fats, at least three times per week. I also use olive oil when I cook, and I try to stick to fats that come from natural sources like egg yolk, almond butter, walnuts on my chicken, etc.

I'll give you more examples later when I show you some different menus you can follow.

Did you know that if you don't eat enough of the good fats, it could elevate your cholesterol? This could lead to heart attacks or other bodily problems like dry hair, dry skin, and brittle nails. You should never completely take out good fat from your nutrition program. Your body needs fat for your hormones and for lubrication of skin, hair, joints, and nails.

I mentioned cholesterol earlier. My clients tell me they always get confused on which is the good cholesterol and which is the bad cholesterol, LDL and HDL. Here is an easy way to remember. LDL is the bad cholesterol. Think of it as "L" for "loser." HDL is the good cholesterol. Think of it as "H" for "happy." See how easy that was? The next time you see your doctor, you'll know what he's talking about when he uses those terms.

8 WHAT'S IN A COMPLETE MEAL? RECAP

So there you have it, nutrition 101 quick and simple! I have found through my clients that the information I have just provided you, and that I have provided to them through the 20 years I've been working, is all they have ever needed to know about nutrition. All the rest is just "mumbo jumbo."

When you sit down to have a meal, you need to identify each of the following. By not eating one of these nutrients, you are robbing your body of the nutrients it needs to look its best and function at its best. Remember: To release the athlete within you, you must feed your machine (your body) and it will respond as predicted.

Just to recap, a "complete meal" should include:

Proteins

Complex Starchy Carbs

Complex Fibrous Carbs

Good Fat

9 I HATE TO COOK

"Not cooking and being prepared ahead of time
are the main reasons most people cannot stick to an eating program."

I REALLY DO NOT LIKE TO COOK. I COOK ALL MY MEALS ON SATURDAY NIGHT AND AGAIN on Wednesday night. The only thing I cook every day is breakfast. I cook my breakfast every night so I can just heat it up at 4:15 in the morning.

Not cooking and being prepared ahead of time are the main reasons most people cannot stick to an eating program. You prepare for your meetings at work. You prepare for your kids' day of school. You plan your weekend activities. You plan your vacations. Why do some of you think you shouldn't have to plan your meals every day? If you don't take care of your health, the rest of the planning that goes on in your life really isn't needed.

So sit down and figure out your meal plans. Spend some time on your health. Clean all the crap (chips, cookies, crackers, cakes, muffins, candies, etc.) out of your pantry. Make a list for the grocery store. It may look like the one on the following page.

Protein: eggs, turkey, fishes, and lean beef

Complex carbs: Uncle Bens™ converted rice, basmati rice, sweet potatoes, yams, cream of rice, slow-cookiing oatmeal, and grits

Simple carbs: sourdough English muffins, Ezekiel bread, pita bread, pasta, tortillas, Kashi GoLean™ cereal, gluten-free pancake mix, granola, and rice cakes

Dairy: low-fat cottage cheese, low-fat plain yogurt (add your own fruit), string cheese, goat cheese (feta), and tofu

Veggies and fruit

Condiments and Flavor Enhancers: low sodium, low in sugar, Mrs. Dash™, cinnamon, garlic, cayenne pepper, rice or soy milk, no-sugar-added apple-sauce, sugar-free maple syrup, low-sugar jelly, almond butter, flax meal

Fats: Extra virgin olive oil, natural peanut butter, almond butter, avocados, olives, balsamic vinegar dressing, walnuts, almonds

And, last but not least, water!!

I usually recommend eight 8-ounce glasses of water per day for an average person who works out in a light-moderate way half an hour a day. For people who are more vigorous in their activities or live in a hot/dry climate, I recommend they drink according to what their body needs. If your mouth becomes dry, you are already beginning to become dehydrated.

I'm sure there are other things you can think of to add to your list. Get creative! Have fun with planning your meals. I tend to eat very boring. I have never liked condiments, and I don't eat dairy. You know, I was the kid who didn't like their foods touching each other. Here are some other tips I have developed through the years to help doctor up healthy food so it is easier to eat.

Doctor up oatmeal or cream of rice:
use sugar-free maple syrup
Add frozen berries
Add dessert baby food
Add peanut butter or almond butter
Add low-sugar jelly
Add walnuts
Add cinnamon
Add rice or soy milk, (vanilla flavored is sweet!)

All of these additions can be used for a variety of things to add flavor without a lot of bad calories. To help your tuna not be so dry, take it out of the can and put it into a container with olive oil on top of it. Leave it overnight or for a half hour or so. The oil seeps through the tuna, giving it flavor and keeping it from being so dry.

Here are some menu samples and some recipes. You can modify the servings in the sample menus to cater to your needs.

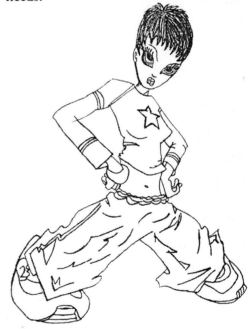

"You need to find the time to cook!"

Meal 1:

3 egg whites/1 whole egg

1 cup of oatmeal

1 cup/piece of fruit

Meal 2:

Turkey sandwich (such as Boars Head™
   low-sodium turkey from the deli)

Ezekiel™ bread, pita bread, or
   sourdough bread

Romaine lettuce

Meal 3:

Chicken breast

1 cup of rice

1 cup of veggies

Meal 4:

1 can of tuna

Sweet potato

2 cups of veggies

Meal 5:

Grilled salmon

Veggie stir fry

Meal 1:

Breakfast wrap (look in recipes)

1 cup of fruit

Meal 2:

Turkey burgers (look in recipes)

2 cup of veggies

Meal 3:

Twice-baked potato (look in recipes)

Meal 4:

Chicken breast

1 cup of rice

2 cups of veggies

Meal 5:

Grilled orange roughy

2 cups of veggies with olive oil

Meal 1:

3 egg whites/ 1 whole egg

1 cup of Kashi GoLean™ cereal

1 cup/piece of fruit

Meal 2:

1 cup of low-fat cottage cheese

1 medium tomato

Meal 3:

Chicken breast

1 cup of pasta

2 cups of veggies

Meal 4:

1 can of tuna

1 cup of rice

2 cups of veggies

Meal 5:

Chicken breast/veggie stir fry

Meal 1:

Protein drink (I like Pro Blend™ or
   Designer Whey™)

Frozen berries and plain yogurt in a
   blender

Meal 2:

3 egg whites/1 whole egg on a sourdough
   English muffin

Low-fat cheese, if desired

Meal 3:

1 golf ball size meatball or meat sauce

1 cup of pasta

2 cups of veggies

Meal 4:

Chicken breast

1 yam

1 cup of veggies

Meal 5:

Flank steak (size of deck of cards)

2 cups of veggies

If you look at each day you can see how I balance out the complex and simple carbs. Remember, simple carbs must be limited throughout your day. For example, if you have bread in the morning then you shouldn't have any the rest of the day, just like I taught my father who previously ate bread at every meal. There are no carbs in the last meal.

By this stage of my book, you should know how to put a meal together. Start with your protein first. Then, if it is not your last meal, decide what type of carb you should have by evaluating how many simple carbs you have already eaten. You should never have more than two meals that contain simple carbs in one day. Remember, eating the complex carbs is how you burn fat. Lastly, pick out your veggies.

Salads are okay but you should also have a hot veggie with it. Salads can make the system slow because it is cold roughage. Women always tell me, "All I eat are salads all day and I haven't dropped a pound." One, they're cold; two, there are no complex or simple carbs; and, three, most people load them up with fatty dressing, cheese, and croutons, and also forget to add protein.

Here is something that always gets laughs out of my clients. Cook fish in your dishwasher. Yes, you read right, your dishwasher. Put your fish with herbs, lemons, limes, etc., in an aluminum foil pouch, pinch tightly, and run it through a cycle of your dishwasher on the top rack. It steams it so good and it keeps your whole place from smelling like fish! You may even wash your dishes at the same time. I developed that because of living in very small apartments and not wanting to smell fish for a week after. I'm serious! Try it!

Now here are a couple of recipes I put together. I don't have a lot; remember, I hate to cook. But these have served me well over the years and my clients all seem to enjoy them.

Oatmeal Pancakes

Crack 4-6 egg whites into a bowl. Slowly pour uncooked, slow-cooking oats into the bowl until you have the consistency of pancake batter.

Add cinnamon to taste.

Pour onto griddle into CD-sized pancakes.

Top off with your favorite topping or eat plain. (Oatmeal pancakes have protein and carbs all in one, perfect for on-the-go people in the morning.)

Breakfast Burrito

3 egg whites/1 whole egg
Breakfast potatoes (hash browns), or you can use Tater Tots.
Low-fat cheese
Tortillas
Salsa

Cook the potatoes until hot. Add eggs and cook. Put into a tortilla with salsa and melted cheese.

Turkey Chili

1 pack extra lean The Turkery Store™ or Jennie-O™ ground turkey
1 14 oz. can dark red kidney beans
1 14 oz. can diced, garlic-stewed tomatoes
Diced celery (optional)
Diced onion (optional)
Chili powder (to taste)

Use 1 tbsp. olive oil in a large pot to soften celery and/or onion first, then add turkey meat.

Cook turkey until broken up and slightly browned.

Add the can of beans and the stewed tomatoes.

Add chili powder. Stir.

Simmer for 30 minutes. (Turkey chili can be eaten alone, on top of rice, or even in a tortilla. This stuff goes a long way!)

4–6 Servings.

Turkey Burgers

1 pack extra-lean The Turkery Store™ or Jennie-O™ ground turkey

1 egg

1 slice of Ezekiel™ bread made into bread crumbs

1 portabella mushroom, diced

1 red pepper, diced

1 Crushed garlic clove

Mix all together in bowl, make patties, and put onto grill.

Makes 4 burgers.

Cajun Fries

4 beaten egg whites

Wedge-cut yams, sweet potatoes, or Idaho potatoes

Cajun seasoning

Ritz™ low-fat crackers (crushed)

Dip wedges into a bowl of egg whites and cajun seasoning (you may also shake the dipped wedges in a plastic bag filled with low-fat, crushed Ritz™ crackers for extra crunch and flavor).

Lay on a baking sheet lightly coated with olive oil.

Bake at 350 degrees for 12-15 min. or until browned to your taste. (Cajun fries are easy, on-the-go complex carbs you can put in a zip baggy and eat in your car with your protein drink. Kids love them!)

Twice-Baked Potatoes

4-6 large Idaho potatoes

Steamed broccoli, chopped

Cooked extra-lean ground turkey breast or chicken breast, diced

Bake the potatoes. When done, cut an oval out of top and scoop out potato into a bowl.

Mix in the broccoli and the meat. Add seasonings, if desired.

Scoop the mixture back into the potato skins. Sprinkle low-fat cheese on top and bake until brown on top or cheese is melted

(Twice-baked potatoes have all the ingredients for a complete meal, perfect for on-the-go lunch people.)

Well, that's about all you're going to get from me when it comes to recipes. I told you, I hate to cook. If you want more ideas, I recommend cookbooks that have gluten-free recipes (a special type of protein that is commonly found in rye, wheat, and barley and can make some people feel bloated and gassy, along with other minor allergic reactions), or Asian stir fry cookbooks. Stick to the healthy cookbooks that focus on natural, unprocessed ingredients. The main thing to remember is to PLAN YOUR MEALS AHEAD OF TIME!

There are companies that cook your food and deliver it right to your door. You tell them what you want and they prepare it for you. It's not cheap, but if that's what it takes to get you to stick to your meals then you need to do it. Your momma's not calling you for dinner anymore! It's up to you to take care of yourself!

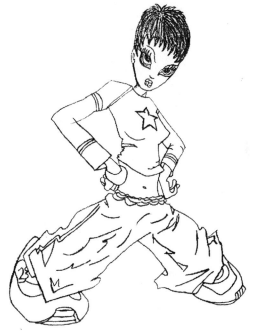

"Cooking in bulk equals... readily available meals!"

10 WHEN I WAS A KID

WHEN I LOOK AT HOW THINGS WERE WHEN I WAS A KID COMPARED TO NOW, I CAN SEE why so many kids and adults struggle with weight problems today. The portions in restaurants have nearly doubled. The public is now allowed to shop where only restaurants or other establishments buy supplies in bulk. Now moms are bringing home giant containers of peanut butter, cookies, chips, etc., to a small family of 4-6 people. This makes everyone eat more because there is more.

SOLUTION: When your family goes to a restaurant, show your kids that their portions should be the size of their fist. Don't make them clean their plates every time they eat. Show them that the portions are smaller on the kids' menu and they could even order an appetizer for a meal. Also, explain that it's okay to take half of their meal home so they can have it for one of their other meals.

SOLUTION: When you bring home large containers of cookies, chips, etc., have your kids help you put the right portion for them into little zip baggies (approximately 1 cup). Then throw the large container away. This way, your kids can grab one little bag to enjoy after school.

There are vending machines in schools. I remember getting excited on "pizza Friday" for lunch. I couldn't have imagined then having vending machines with real junk food in them for us! Only the teachers' lounge had vending machines. My mom never allowed us to just sit and eat junk food. I remember when my brother grabbed a bag of chips and headed to his room, she would say, "Put them back unless you eat some real food with them. Like, make a turkey sandwich or something with some substance to it." Then she always finished with, "You're not going to sit around and eat junk all day!"

SOLUTION: Teach your kids which foods are better to pick if they end up eating something out of a vending machine. For example, pretzels, baked chips, and granola bars are better choices then cheese puffs and candy.

SOLUTION: Teach your kids what "a complete meal" is. They must always have a protein, a starchy carbohydrate, and fibrous carbohydrate. Have them make a small sandwich, to go with the little bag of chips they grabbed; have some cut up fruit and veggies already in little bags, also. Ask them to help you prepare their little baggies. They love to learn and help out!

No one takes time to eat right anymore. I understand the world moves a lot faster now compared to back when I was a kid, but you still have to take care of yourself. Even when it comes to being active, people will say they don't have time.

SOLUTION: If your kids see you taking the time to take care of yourself, they will learn and follow your example. Show them how important it is to get the right foods all day. Let them help you buy groceries and prepare in bulk so that you have all your little meals ready and accessible. They will be so ahead of the game once they become adults, living on their own.

SOLUTION: I didn't have a cell phone or a computer when I was a kid. I had to ride my bike to be able to talk to my friends. Show your kids that you can take the stairs instead of the escalator or elevator whenever they are available. You can park farther away from the building so that you will get some exercise just walking to your destination. Play active games like Twister™, put some music on and DANCE! They'll love it! Being active is so important for your health.

I also had gym class every day all 12 years of school! You have no idea how that one period of gym class every day for 12 years could change your kids' health. I know, I know, they've cut out a lot of extracurricular classes in our school systems. Well, I don't consider our kids' health and well-being as extracurricular. So we've got more food and less activity, which spells weight problems.

SOLUTION: Teach your kids early how to exercise and stretch. In the chapter, "If You Don't Use It, You Lose It," in PART II, which comes next, I have some great exercises you and your kids can do together. There are no weights involved, only a rubber band and a physio ball. Kids under 12 should not use weights. My program only takes 20–30 minutes, max! Your kids are never too young to learn! Just think of the great habits you will be instilling in them!

You need to take responsibility for your health and set an example for your family. Teach your kids about nutrition. It's so easy! I just taught you everything you need to know in basic, easy terminology. Make your kids help you prepare meals ahead of time. They'll need to do it someday, unless you plan on them living with you forever. I can't believe how many teens I have trained who are heading off to college and don't even know how to boil an egg, or even water for that matter!

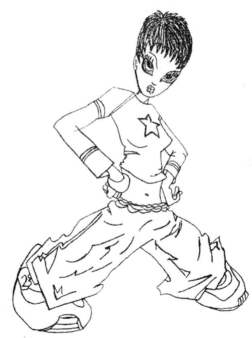

**"Healthy kids equals...
healthy adults!"**

On the following pages, write what your eating habits were when you were a kid. What emotions were involved, if any? Now write what habits you are creating or passing on to your kids.

90 DAYS TO A NEW YOU

PART II

Exercises With Illustrations

11 IF YOU DON'T USE IT, YOU LOSE IT

"The way you live your life, the perspective you select,
is a choice you make every single day when you wake up.
It's yours to decide."
–Lance Armstrong

THAT QUOTE IS SO TRUE. IT DOESN'T MATTER WHAT AGE YOU ARE, IF YOU KEEP using your muscles, they will keep performing for you. By exercising, you will improve strength, flexibility, and coordination.

Within The Angela Jordan System, I have developed my workout system. My type of workout regimen is called Functional Freestyle Fitness. Functional means using the body to do the move without relying on a machine. Freestyle means using the upper and lower body at the same time.

By doing my workout, you will have great results faster with less time invested. I believe in quality not quantity. I also believe in doing a variety of movements to keep the body from falling into a plateau.

Regardless of their age, I have made all of my clients do exercises they thought their body would never be able to do.

Kids are great to work with because they have no fears or boundaries on what they are willing to try. Developing strength, coordination, and flexibility at a young age really puts you ahead of the game once you start aging and the body starts to lose these qualities. Usually between the ages of 35 to 45 you will notice your body losing muscle tone and strength, coordination and flexibility.

I have helped a lot of kids improve in sports, gain confidence, and improve their self-esteem within themselves and their bodies. My workout is great for

ents would rather use weights than those strong little bands.

We all know that as we get older we can start to develop fears and boundaries when it comes to our body. The problem with this is, every day I see people come into my gym dealing with weaknesses, lack of coordination, and instability in their bodies because of these fears and boundaries they have developed.

You should train your muscles to work and react the way you need them to in every day life.

kids of all ages. Generally, kids under 12 should not use weights. Rubber bands are a great way to substitute weights so that they may still strengthen their bodies in a safe, effective way. Bands come in all lengths and thicknesses which results in different strengths of resistance. Some have handles and others are just a flat piece of rubber. I prefer handles for better comfort and control. Those bands aren't as easy as they look. Sometimes, my cli-

You must focus on being positive and push yourself to help your body function at its best. I have clients in their 70s who could hardly walk up the stairs by themselves. After doing my workout program twice a week for 30 minutes for only four weeks, they were not only able to easily climb the stairs, but also jump on a trampoline! As long as you have no fears or boundaries, your muscles can strengthen and learn to do anything. The younger you are when you start working out, the easier it will be for you as the body does its usual aging process. But also remember, you are never too old to get started! Come on, the athlete within you is just waiting to be released!

Because I have been working out for 32 years, since the age of five, and I have experienced several different types of workouts, I have picked out four exercises per body part that I feel every body should be able to perform at any age. There are several exercise routines you can do but that's for my next book. Stay tuned!

I have put a little program together that allows you to have variety by letting you pick your exercises for that body part. I also made sure to maximize your time with quality instead of quantity. So your workout should take only 20 minutes, 30 minutes, max in case you need a longer rest period in between exercises. Remember, more is not always better!

The three things you will need to focus on to guarantee a great workout are form, tempo, and intensity level. Without proper form, you will fail to work the intended muscles and risk injury in the process. Without the right tempo (speed) during your repetitions, you will fail to work the muscle to its full potential. Without the proper intensity level, you will not have an effective workout.

Your form is so important. If you're not working the right muscle, why bother? I drive all my clients crazy because I am constantly on them about their form, yet they always tell me that if they didn't work out with me, they would end up throwing their back out. Every time I walk into a gym, I see people using too heavy weights and swinging them around with improper form. Avoid getting sloppy, watch your form.

Tempo is another one that everyone has an opinion on. I believe in doing what your body does naturally with everyday life tasks. You should train your muscles to work and react the way you need them to in everyday life. If you train a muscle to contract slowly on the move, you are training it to move slowly and have a bad reaction time. This is where I get people who lift really slowly all the time and then they try to take something out of the trunk of their car that is heavy, the object slips, their muscles can't react quickly enough, and they pull their muscles, injuring themselves. If you put a huge bodybuilder who trains slowly and for size in a ring with a boxer who trains for strength and speed, it doesn't matter how much bigger the bodybuilder is than the boxer, the boxer will get a couple hits on the bodybuilder before he even tries to throw a punch. As you can see, their muscles are trained for their type of sport. So make sure you train your muscles for the type of activities you expect them to perform.

As far as tempo, I prefer you use the tempo you use in everyday life. When you contract the muscle, you count two seconds, which means you move quickly. When you come out of the repetition or, as we say, you do the negative part of the move, you count 3-4 seconds. Once you get to the end of the negative, you explode right back into contracting it again, no break between repetitions. You basically get into a rhythm, or a perfect tempo.

When I talk about intensity, I mean the amount of effort you are giving to your workout. If you don't push yourself and, instead, just go through the moves with little to no effort, then you will not see very good results from your workout program. The following page explains what you should experience at each level of intensity. It also gives which intensity level you should use during each stage of your workout. Additional information about the workout follows on the graph on page 74.

I have listed four exercises per body part with the exception of shoulders. Because the shoulder muscles are smaller muscles and assist during chest and back exercises, you only have to pick one exercise from the two exercises I have given you for each muscle. The shoulder is comprised of three muscles: front deltoid (anatomical term for shoulder), medial (middle) deltoid, and rear deltoid. I have also put together four ab routines. Pick one routine per workout and do the entire routine from start to finish, as I have written it.

My workout program spans 90 days which can be performed with my 90-Day Detox. It is important to understand that physical activity is needed for health and well-being and will speed up the results of any nutrition program. My 90-Day Detox program will work with not only the workout program I have developed, but also any other physical activity you choose to incorporate. My 90-Day Detox program will be explained in detail later in PART III.

In the first 30 days, you will be performing each exercise for 30 seconds. In weeks one and two, you will do a level 5 intensity. Week three, you will do a level 7 intensity and week four, you will do a level 9 intensity for the whole 30 seconds. Your rest periods between each exercise should be 30 seconds during all three months. When performing exercises that require doing one side and then the other, you will do each side equally for the entire time.

In the second 30 days, you will perform each exercise for 45 seconds. In week one, you will do a level 5 intensity. In weeks two and three, you will do a level 7 intensity. In week four, you will do a level 9 intensity for the whole 45 seconds.

In the final 30 days, you will perform each exercise for 60 seconds. In week one, you will do a level 5 intensity. In week two, you will do a level 7 intensity. In weeks three and four, you will do a level 9 intensity for the whole 60 seconds.

Try to keep your rest periods between each exercise at 30 seconds. If you notice that you're still breathing too heavily after 30 seconds of rest because you just did a level 9 intensity, then give yourself an extra 10-15 seconds of rest before you start the next exercise. By doing this type of workout you are getting some cardio training along with your resistance (weights and/or rubber bands) training.

Once you have finished the 90-day program, you may continue with the same program using the intensity level and exercise workout time that best suits your physical abilities. For example, if you're not feeling physically up to working out, yet you still want to make the body move and loosen up, then you can do your exercises for only 30 seconds, performing a level 5 intensity. If you are physically athletically fit, then you can do your exercises at a level 9 intensity for any of the time frames depending on how much time you have and how quick you want to see results with your body.

For timesaving reasons, I have put together five multimuscle movement exercises for a quick, fullbody workout. Perform each exercise for 30 seconds at a level 7-9 intensity and rest for 30-45 seconds between each exercise. Push yourself and have fun with these, they are not easy!

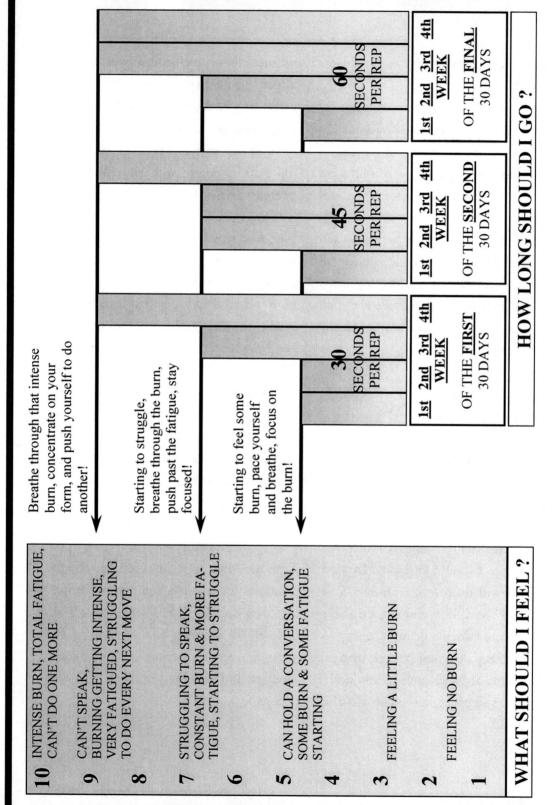

WORKOUT INTENSITY GUIDE

WHAT SHOULD I FEEL ?

10 INTENSE BURN, TOTAL FATIGUE, CAN'T DO ONE MORE

9 CAN'T SPEAK, BURNING GETTING INTENSE, VERY FATIGUED, STRUGGLING TO DO EVERY NEXT MOVE

8

7 STRUGGLING TO SPEAK, CONSTANT BURN & MORE FATIGUE, STARTING TO STRUGGLE

6

5 CAN HOLD A CONVERSATION, SOME BURN & SOME FATIGUE STARTING

4 FEELING A LITTLE BURN

3

2 FEELING NO BURN

1

Breathe through that intense burn, concentrate on your form, and push yourself to do another!

Starting to struggle, breathe through the burn, push past the fatigue, stay focused!

Starting to feel some burn, pace yourself and breathe, focus on the burn!

HOW LONG SHOULD I GO ?

1st 2nd 3rd 4th WEEK OF THE FIRST 30 DAYS	1st 2nd 3rd 4th WEEK OF THE SECOND 30 DAYS	1st 2nd 3rd 4th WEEK OF THE FINAL 30 DAYS
30 SECONDS PER REP	**45** SECONDS PER REP	**60** SECONDS PER REP

How often should you work out? A lot depends on your individual recovery time. Most of my clientele work out twice a week with me for 30 minutes at a level 7-9 intensity. I have a couple of athletic clients who can work out three times a week for 30 minutes each at a level 7-9 intensity. If you still feel too sore to work out a day or two after your workout, then give your body an extra day to recover. I can't sat this enough, more is not always better!

The two biggest mistakes are: cutting too much food and doing too much cardio.

I always get the question, "How much cardio should I do?" I have watched so many people make the same mistake over and over when it comes to trying to lose weight and get in shape. The two biggest mistakes are: cutting too much food and doing too much cardio.

Weights and/or rubber band training will shape your body and speed up your metabolism faster than any running/cardio workout will. Don't worry ladies, you don't have to get big and bulky to speed up your metabolism, you just need to tone what you've got. You've seen it, the person who comes to the gym religiously every day, going on the same treadmill, running on it for an hour at a level 9-10 every time, sweating like crazy, yet their body never looks real lean and toned, and their body doesn't really change much. This is because they are doing too much cardio for the type of nutrition they are taking in and they are probably slacking in the resistance training department.

You can not trick the body! No matter how much you run, if you don't get enough of the right food, for the amount of running you are doing, your body will sacrifice muscle before it will burn body fat. Yes, I am serious! Your body will hold body fat so you don't pass out on that treadmill. That's why these people look loose and soft and they do not hold a lot of lean muscle mass. A true runner eats a lot of calories! They have to so they can keep lean mass and low body fat so their bodies run like a cheetah.

If you are going to run, I suggest you run in intervals where you do a medium run and then do sprints. By sprinting, you engage your butt and hamstrings, which in turn protects your knees and low back from impact. When you do a slow jog the whole time, you do a lot of unnecessary pounding on all of the joints in the body.

You must have your resistance training and nutrition dialed in before you add in the amount of cardio you do. Cardio is the last thing I add into a client's workout. I get them on my fitness program first, which is fast-paced, and introduces them into my nutrition program, and then if they want to come in even leaner, I

Once my weight training and my nutrition were locked in and I had done as much as I could with my body, I added cardio and locked in my results! It works every time!

Cardio is used for the cardiovascular system which includes your heart, your lungs, and your circulatory system.

Cardio will improve the function and efficiency of all of these You will also burn fat, if done correctly. I recommend

Your resistance training, your nutrition and your cardio, have to all be in sync for your body to be at its best.

add some kind of cardio. No, it's not running. I prefer jumping jacks and jumping on a trampoline, which has no impact. Your resistance training, your nutrition, and your cardio, all have to be in sync for your body to be at its best.

When I was in competition, cardio was my last secret weapon, added in after I had already exhausted my resources for weights and nutrition. I would add a step mill and/or a treadmill for 30 minutes.

that you do cardio for 20-30 minutes, max, and that you do intervals, which I'll explain in a moment. Doing intervals helps you burn fat quicker. You know how when you first get on a treadmill and you feel a bit winded and cranky and feel like you physically can't do it? Once you stay on for a few minutes and the intensity level hasn't changed, you notice it's not so bad. This means your heart has gotten used to what you are doing, so you can kick it up a notch with your intensity level. Remember, you don't want to stay at that high intensity level for too long because you will no longer burn fat and switch over to burning hard-earned muscle!

Changing your intensity levels back and forth challenges the body to pull from the fat storages yet doesn't push it past its limits to where it goes after your muscle mass.

=====

If you're not seeing results in the first month, check your intensity levels during your workout.

=====

The intervals look like this: 3-5 minute warmup, level 5 intensity; the next minute go the whole minute at a level 9, really push it! After that minute, go back to the level 5 for 30 seconds only. If you still have trouble talking after these 30 seconds, give yourself an extra 15 seconds. Now go the next minute back up to the level 9 intensity. Continue these intervals, leaving a couple of minutes to cool down at the end. The type of machine and or bands you use will determine what "number" level you use for that particular machine. The intensity levels I mentioned, levels 5 and 9, go by your personal intensity level, like in my graph on page 74.

Concentrate on your resistance training program and nutrition first. Add your cardio when you need to kick it up a notch. If you're not seeing results in the first month, check your intensity levels during your workout. Make sure you're giving it all you've got. If those are good then check your nutrition. Remember, if you don't eat unhealthy food then you won't have to burn off unhealthy food. As I always say to my clients, "If you don't put it in your mouth, you won't have to work it off!"

Now conquer those fears, lose those boundaries, and let's get that body moving!!

Pick one exercise per body part (group) and one full ab routine per workout.

Refer to the Intensity Workout Chart on page 74.

Add cardio as needed.

To see demonstrations of the rubber
band work out, logon to:

www.NinetyDaysToANewYou.com

EXERCISES

JUMPING JACKS

Start at 30 seconds and work up to five minutes straight. Jumping Jacks pump the lymph system (a network of vessels that transport water and minerals around the body) in the armpits and groin area (crease of the legs in the front.) A better lymph system equals better fat loss.

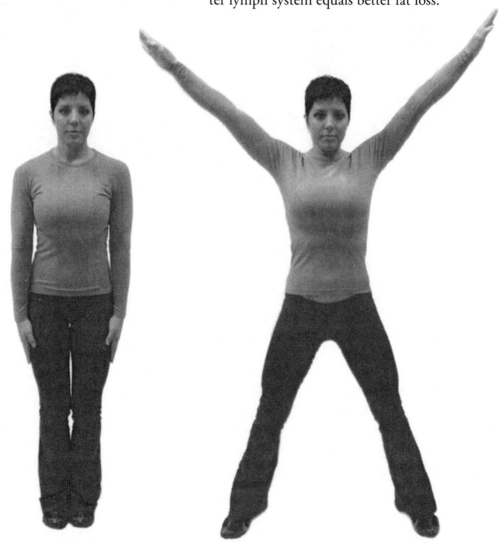

PUSH-UPS

These are pretty much self-explanatory. Keep your bellybutton pulled in to support your low back, move the body like it's a board. Go to your knees if you feel it in your low back. Exhale as you come up. Hands should be far enough apart so when you lower yourself your bent elbows do not stick out past your wrists.

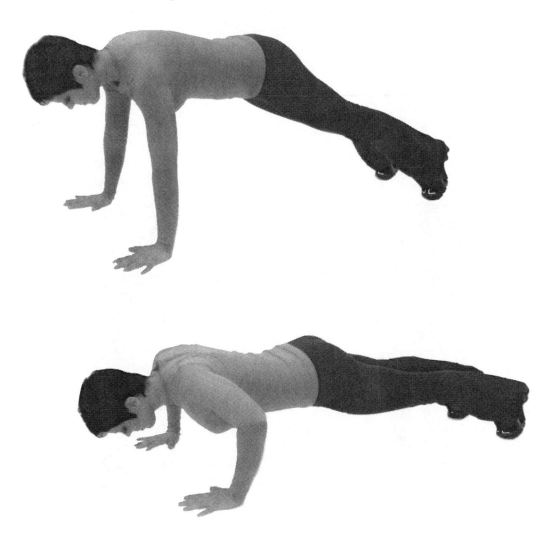

STANDING FLIES WITH BAND

Stand on band with both feet, feet are hip width apart. Bring your arms up like you are going to hug a big tree. Keep your bellybutton pulled into the spine and avoid arching back during the movement. Bring your hands up to face level, touching pinky fingers together and act like you're holding a bowl in the air to get a full squeeze of the chest muscles.

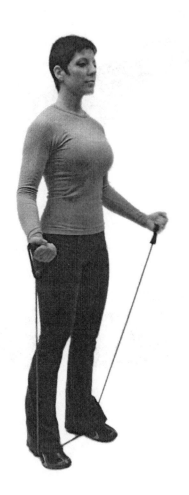
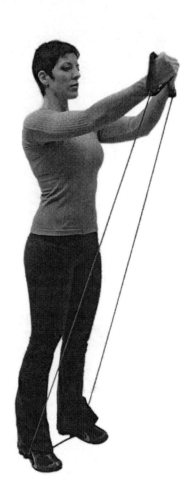

ONE-LEG PUSH-UPS

Same as the PUSH-UP only now you will hold one leg up while you do reps of 10, and then switch to other leg. Keep going until your time is up. Engage your butt muscle to hold your leg up and out straight. Really pull your bellybutton in to support your low back. If you feel it in your low back, it means you're not pulling your bellybutton in tight enough.

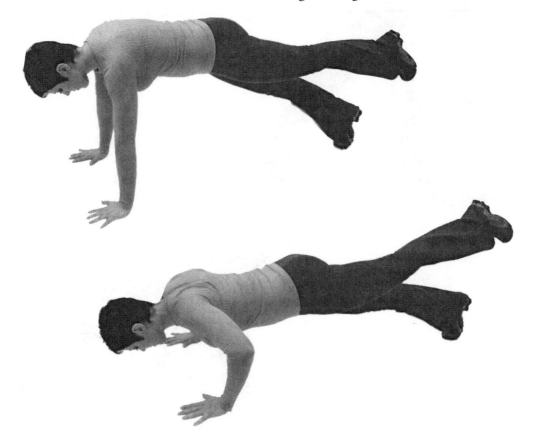

PUSH-UPS ON THE PHYSIO BALL

(A physio ball is a large, inflatable rubber ball used for balance training.) You can either do an incline push-up with your hands on the ball and feet on the floor, or do a decline push-up with your feet on the ball and your hands on the floor. Really engage your abs by pulling your bellybutton in and keeping the whole body tight and straight like a board. Keep your butt level with your head so that you don't sink into your low back.

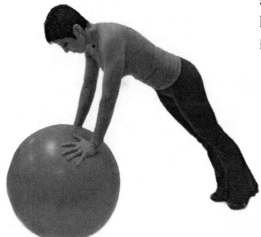

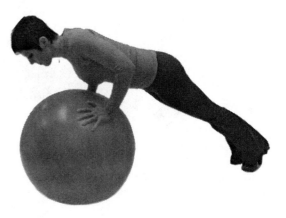

SEATED ROW

Pull your shoulder blades together and stick your chest out. Exhale when you pull back. Hand positions can be with thumbs up and/or palms up to work a lower part of the back.

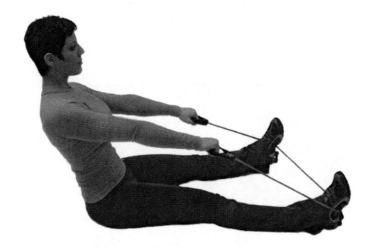

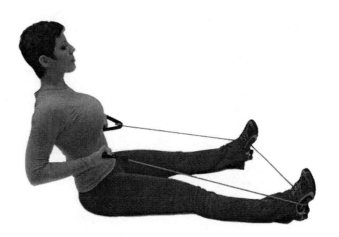

ONE-ARM ROWS

Standing in a lunge with the band under the front foot, lean your elbow on your knee, keeping your back straight. Do not round your back outward or hunch over. Pull the band with one hand like you're trying to start a lawn mower. Keep your abs pulled in and try to bring your elbow back toward the side of your body each time you pull back. You will do the full time on each side.

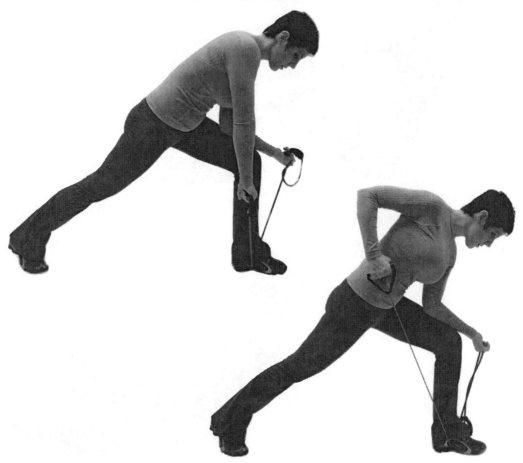

BENT-OVER RAISES

With both feet on the band, standing with feet hip width apart, cross the handles to the opposite hands. Bend over with a flat back, not rounded, and pull your abs in. Pull the handles out to the sides and back at the same time, keeping arms slightly bent as if you were pushing people away from you. Squeeze your shoulder blades together with each pullback.

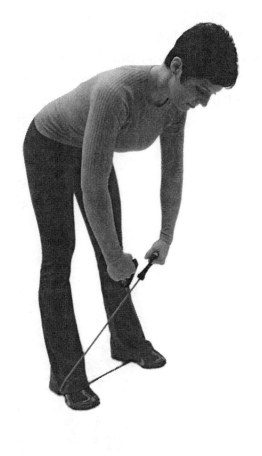
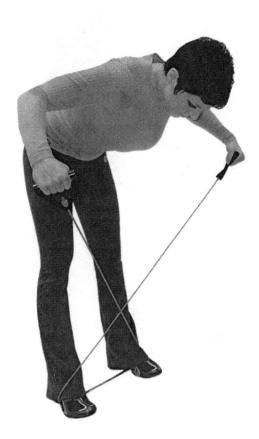

PULL DOWNS OR PULL APARTS

If you have a door or something you can put the band over, you may do pull downs. Keep abs pulled in and pull the band down by pushing your shoulder blades down and back, picture jabbing your elbows into your sides. The move mimics that of pulling your arms down as if someone were trying to tickle under your arms. To do pull aparts, you will hold the band above the head and pull away from each end as you take the band behind the head. You may also hold one arm straight and pull the other arm down and away to do one side at a time.

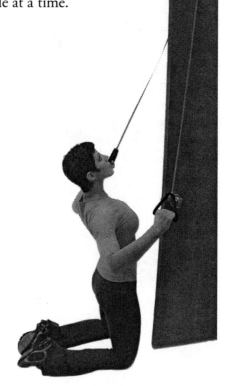

SQUAT

Stay on your heels with toes relaxed as you pull your bellybutton in to support your low back. Exhale as you come up. Stick butt back like you are going to sit in a chair, then thrust hips forward to stand up.

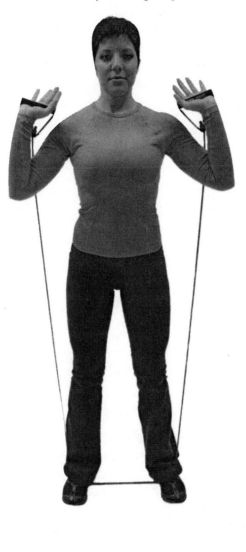

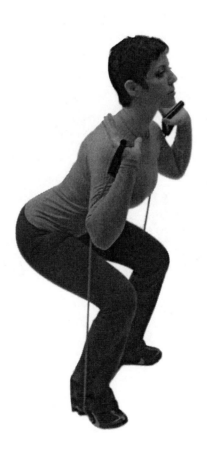

STATIC LUNGE

Step way back, making sure your front knee does not come over your front foot when you lunge down. Pull your bellybutton in, push through your heel in the front—not your toes—bend your back knee first like you were kneeling down and then straighten the legs at the same time. Remember to keep your chest up and exhale as you come up.

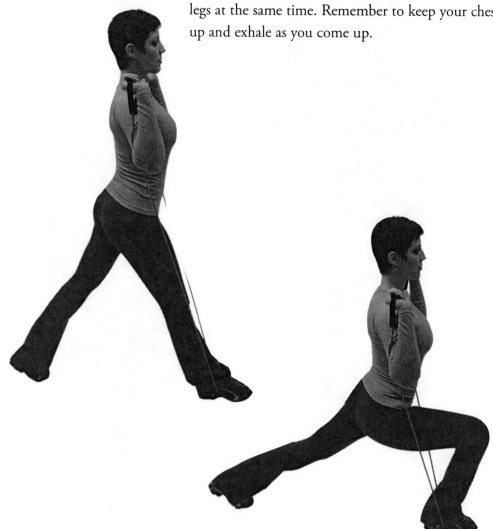

SUMO JUMPS/ SUMO SQUAT

Using a very wide stance, stay on your heels, sit your butt back, pull your bellybutton in, and exhale as you come up. When jumping, act as if you are sitting in a chair, then thrust hips to come up. Raise arms as you jump up.

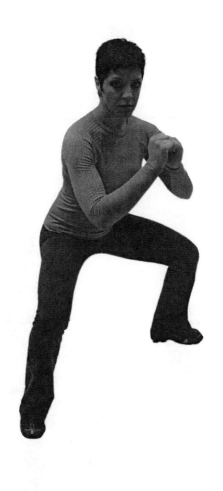

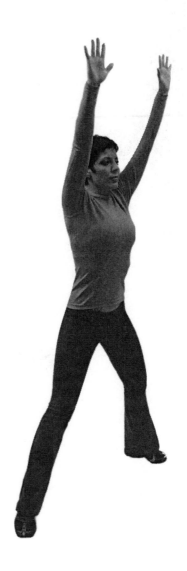

WALKING LUNGES

When you step forward, land on your front heel first, bend the back knee right into a lunge, push through your front heel to come up—not your toes. Keep your chest up at all times, do not use your back. Exhale as you come up.

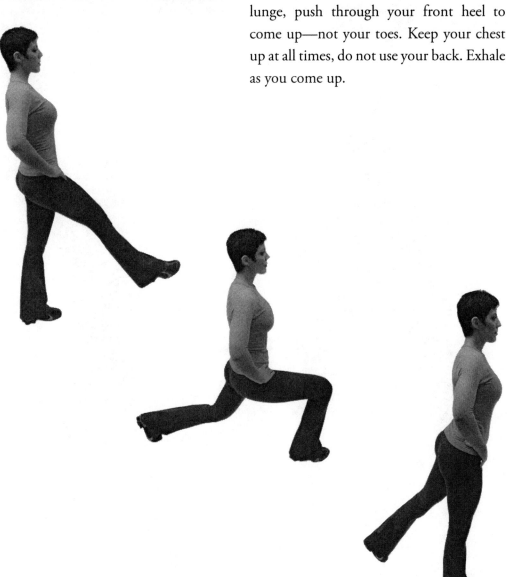

ABOVE THE HEAD PRESS

With both feet on the band and abs pulled in, push the band above your head, avoiding arching the back. You may also sit on a ball to do this.

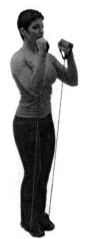

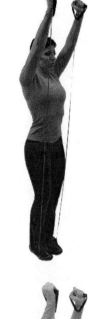

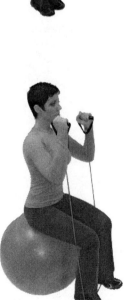

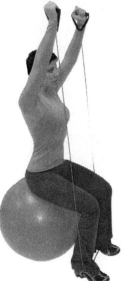

FRONT RAISES

With both feet on the band, lift band in front of you with straight arms. You may do one at a time or both at the same time, with your hand position in "holding a can" position.

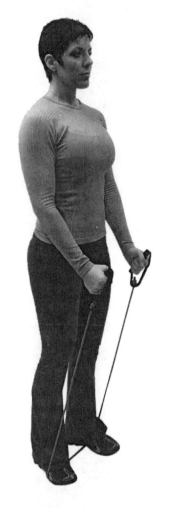

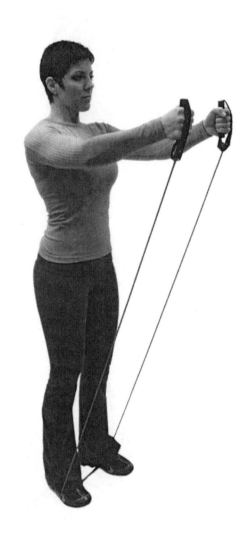

LATERAL RAISE

Lead with your elbows and make hands level with elbows—not higher. Act like you are pushing people away from you. Exhale as you come up.

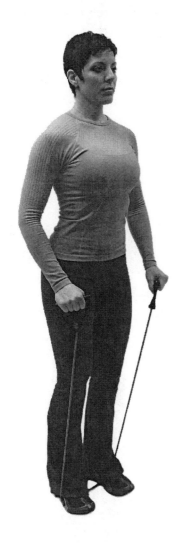
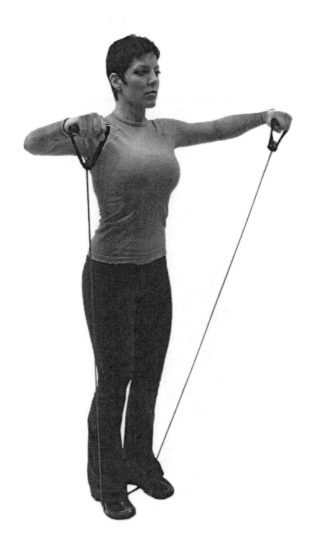

UPRIGHT ROWS

Same as a LATERAL RAISE only now you pull the band up in front of the body, up to the middle of the chest. Keep first fingers touching each other the whole time as you pull and direct your elbows up first, making a "V" at the top of the move. Pretend like you are making an arc in front of the body while you are pulling up, as if you are tracing a big belly on the front of you. Keep abs pulled in and avoid arching in the low back as you pull.

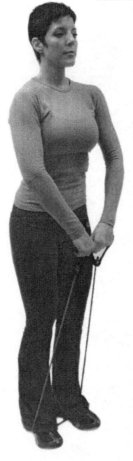
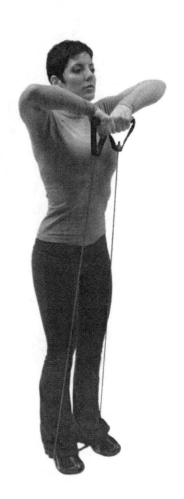

ONE~ARM FLASHERS

Either wrap a band around a door knob or hold a band in one hand while you rotate other arm. Keep your arm bent at 90 degrees and close to the body. Rotate your arm out like you are flashing someone with that side of your shirt. When coming back, stop movement at 90 degrees to the body. Do not bring your arm all the way back into the body so as not to lose the tension on the band.

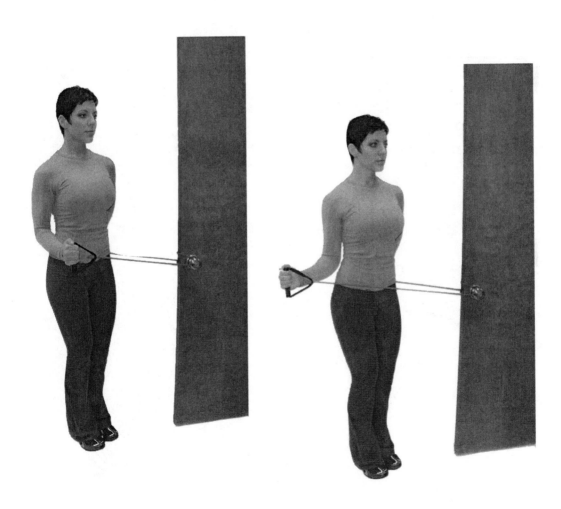

TOUCHDOWN PULLS

Seated on a ball, both feet on the band, cross the handles in the opposite hands. Then pull the band up and back, squeezing your shoulder blades together and sticking your chest out, ending with your elbows bent and looking like you're signaling for a touchdown.

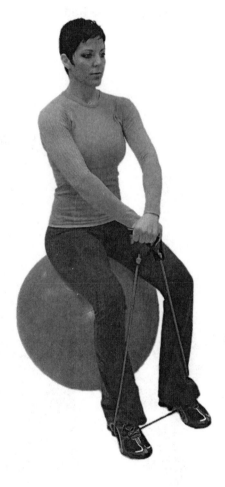

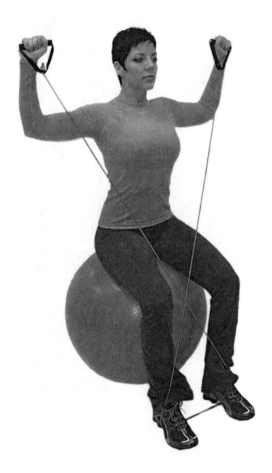

TRICEP PUSH-DOWNS

Keep your shoulders back and chest out. Once you push down, only come back to a 90-degree angle at the elbow. Exhale as you push down. Keep your bellybutton pulled in to support your low back.

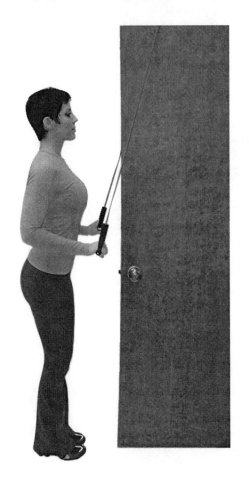
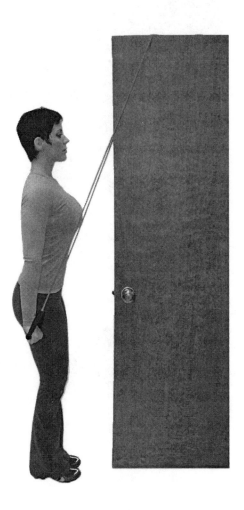

TRICEP PUSH-UPS

Hands below chest, your elbows run into the ribs as you come down. Keep them in tight as you push up. Do not arch the back.

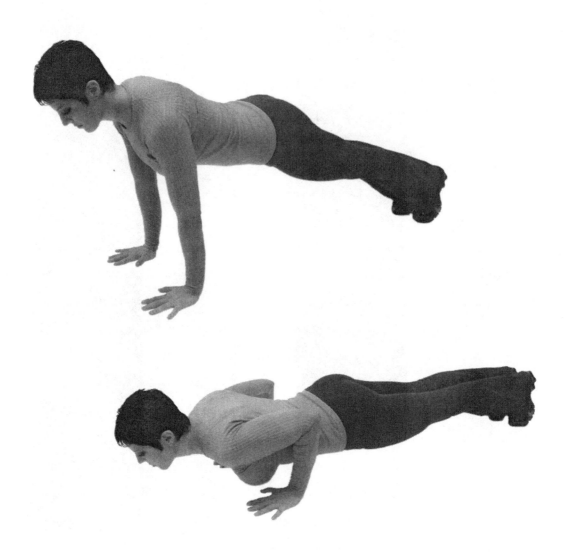

OVERHEAD EXTENSIONS

Put a band on your back foot and lunge forward on your front foot. With the band behind you, bring your hands up to the ceiling, keeping your elbows close to your ears. Bend your elbows, dropping the band back, and then straighten your arms to pull the band back up. Do not arch during this exercise. Pull your bellybutton in.

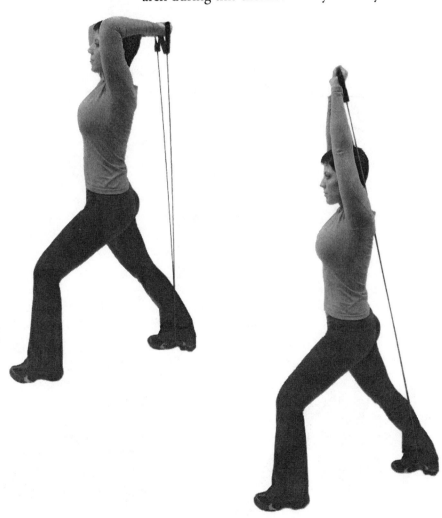

KICKBACKS

Seated on a ball or standing with the band under both feet, start with bent arms and the handles at your hips. Push the handles back behind you, squeezing the back of the arms. Do not move the whole arm, only bend and straighten the bottom part of the arm, keeping the shoulders back and in place. Keep your abs pulled in to support the back.

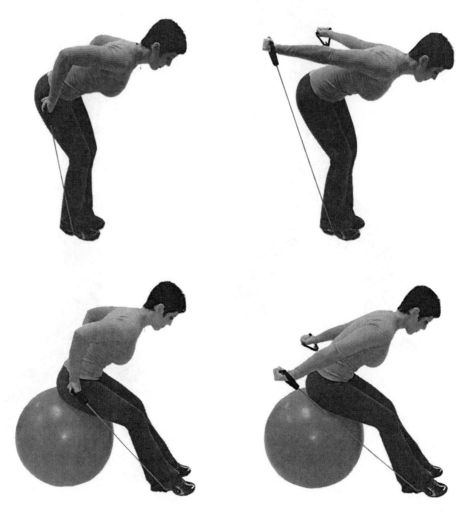

STANDING CURLS

Keep chest up, bellybutton pulled in, exhale as you curl up. Control the move going down, don't let your elbows snap down. Don't arch your back and yank the resistance up.

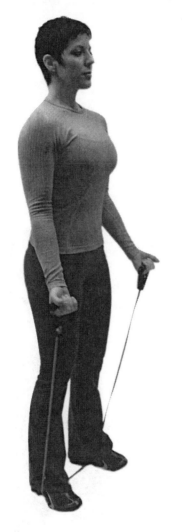

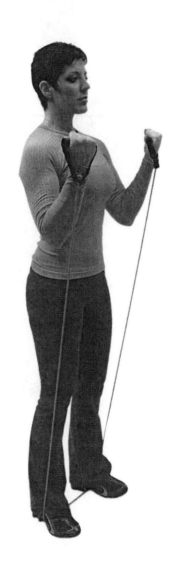

HAMMER CURLS

Standing with both feet on the band, curl the band across the body in front of you, one at a time, with palms facing in toward the body.

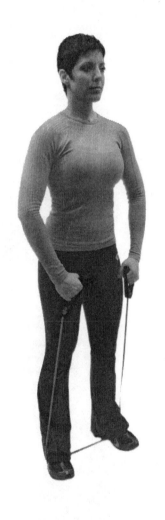

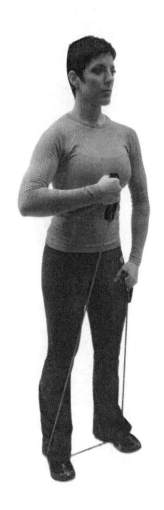

OUT TO SIDE SEATED CURLS

Sitting on a ball, band under widely spread feet, curl the band out to the sides of your body. Sit up straight, abs pulled in. Pull up quick and let down slower.

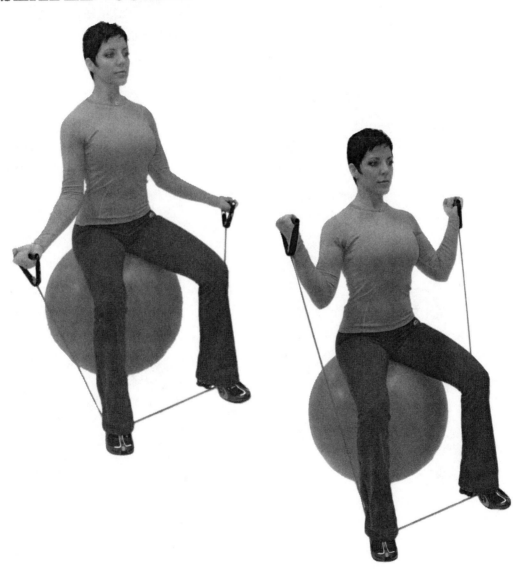

AGAINST THE WALL CURLS

Lean against the wall, band under feet, feet out away from wall so the body is at an angle. Keep your elbows against the wall the whole time you curl the band. This mimics the incline curl, which is when you lie on a bench that is inclined, letting your arms hang down and back, then curling your lower arm up while keeping your upper arm back.

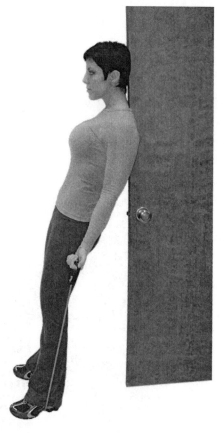
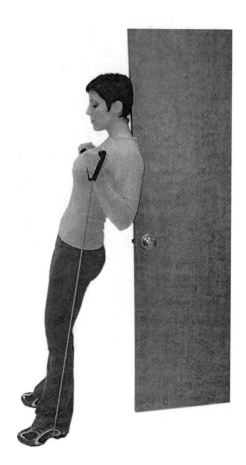

LOW AB STRADDLE "V"-UPS

Keep your arms straight and push away from what you're holding, to avoid pulling with your biceps. Keep your legs in a wide "V" and very straight through the whole exercise. If you have a tight low back, slightly bend your knees and don't pull your legs up as high. Bring feet toward armpits.

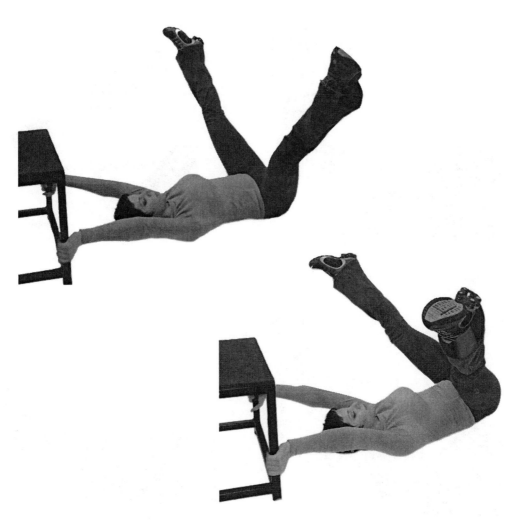

OBLIQUE PIKE-UPS

You are making a "V" in the air with your legs by keeping feet together and pulling legs from one armpit and down and up to the other armpit and down. Hold a pillow or book between the feet or knees during the exercise to engage the low abs more.

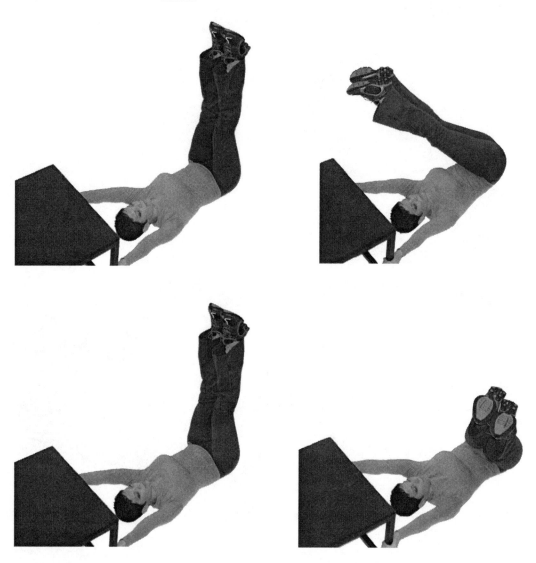

PIKE-UPS

Same as OBLIQUE PIKE-UPS only you will just pull the legs straight up to chest or chin.

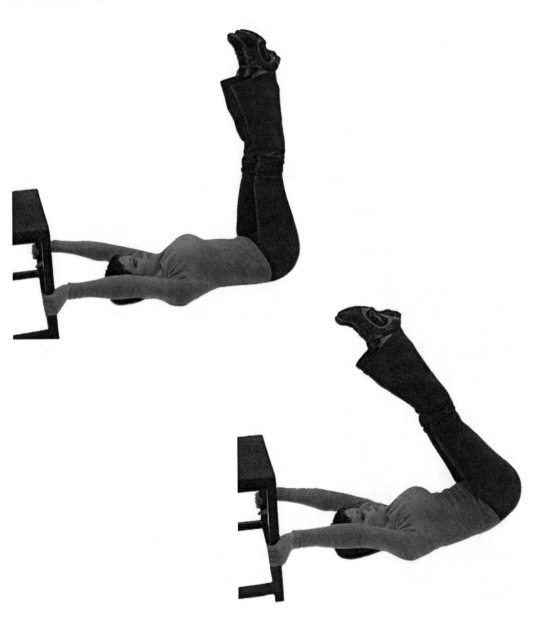

OBLIQUE DOWN TO THE SIDE ALTERNATES

Make sure you twist in waist when your legs go down to the side. One leg should be on top of the other. Exhale as you pull the legs up using your side abs, not pulling with your back. Try to push your back down to the floor as you crunch your side abs and pull your legs up.

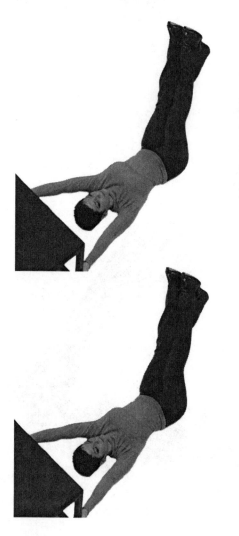
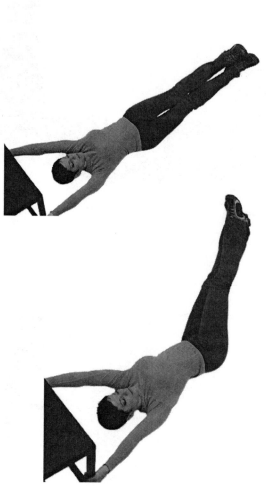

SIDE CRUNCHES

Keep your chin up so you engage the abs and avoid pulling on your neck. By turning your leg out, you disengage your hip flexors (a muscle which attaches under the front hip bones, goes through the midbody and attaches to your lower spinal area) and concentrate more on your abs.

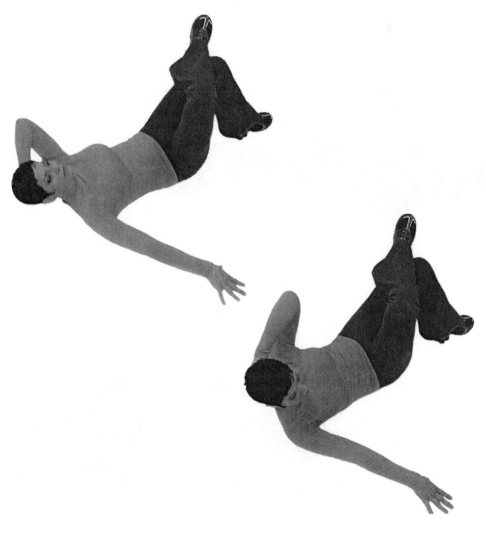

FROG-LEG CRUNCHES

Keep your chin up, never interlock your fingers behind your head, keep your elbows open or just reach with your hands to the ceiling. Squeeze your butt and push your knees to the floor during the whole exercise.

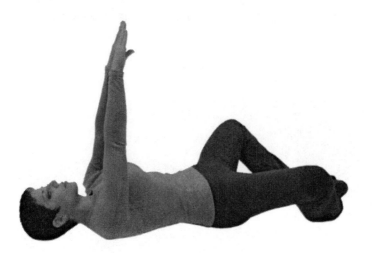

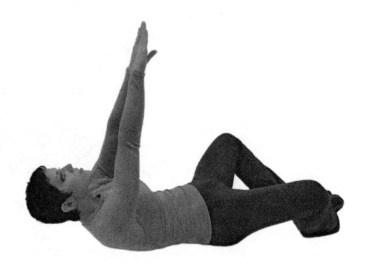

GOLF TWIST WITH ROPE

Keep your arms locked straight. Keep the abs pulled in and avoid arching into your back. Swing up quick and let the band down slower.

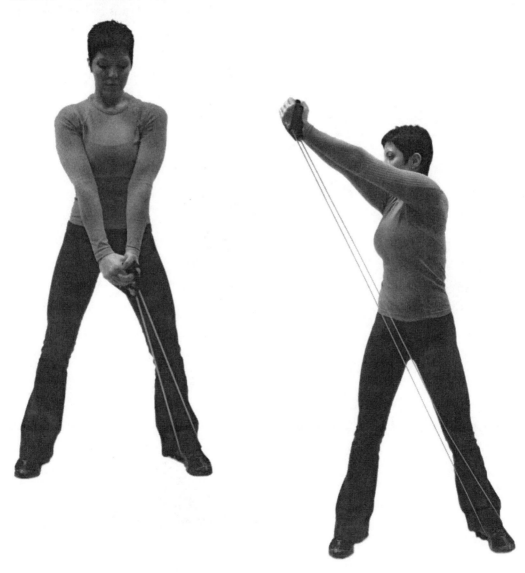

PENDULUM

Keep your legs at 90 degrees to your hips. Think of pulling your feet toward your hand as you go side to side. Really concentrate on using your side abs to pick up the legs, not your low back. If you feel it in your back, don't drop your legs as low. Keep the palms of your hands facing the ceiling, don't use your arms to help you.

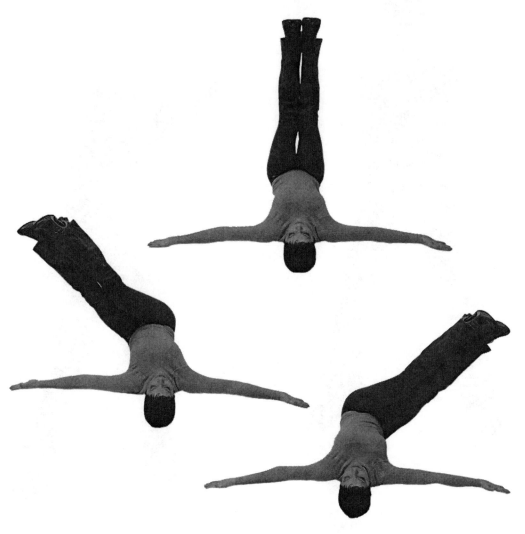

REVERSE PIKE CRUNCHES

Hold a throw pillow or magazine in your hands above your face. Bring your feet to the object. Do not move the object toward your feet. Lift your tailbone off the floor every time, and avoid swinging the legs past the 90 degrees of the hips so you do not go into your low back.

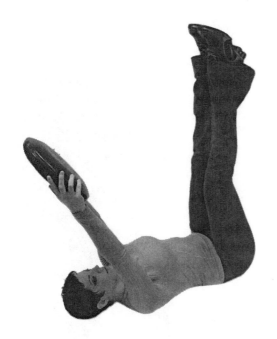

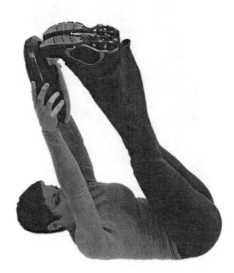

PIKE CRUNCHES

By holding something between your feet you will engage the lower abs more. Keep your chin up and reach for the object.

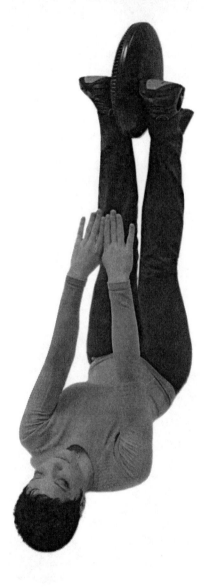

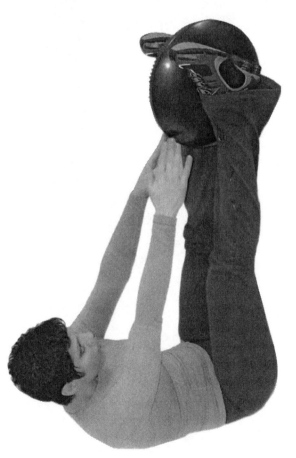

PIKE CRUNCHES /REACH SIDE TO SIDE

Same as PIKE CRUNCHES only you will reach both hands to one side of object and then down and then back up on the other side.

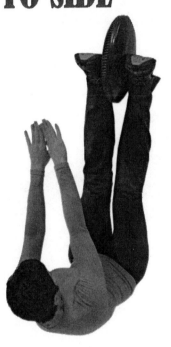

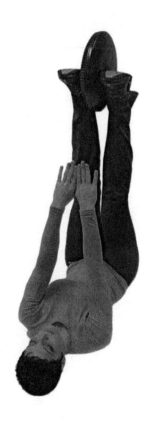

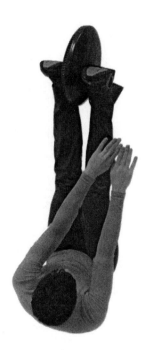

PLANK KNEE PULLS

Make sure you really try to pull your knee to the opposite elbow. Your body will need to hunch up like a cat to pull your knee up to the elbow, and then you will return flat to a plank position once you bring your leg back down.

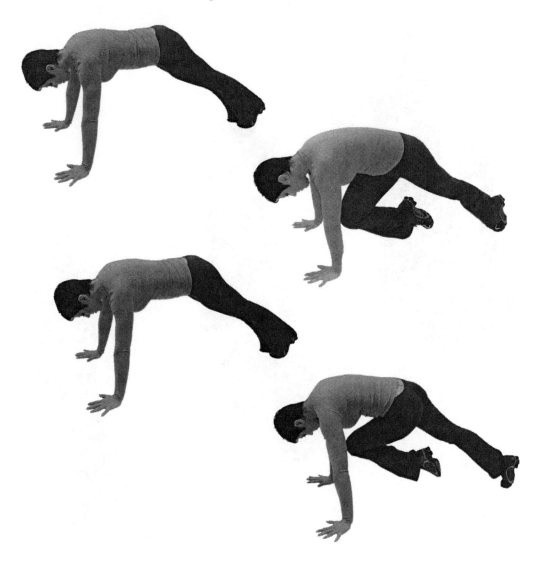

ELBOW PLANK HOLD WITH ALTERNATING FEET

Make sure you keep your legs locked straight and lift them back and forth at a normal pace, keeping your bellybutton pulled in real tight and your butt tucked under (kind of like what a dog does when it gets in trouble). If you feel this in your low back, you're not pulling your bellybutton in and keeping your butt tucked under enough.

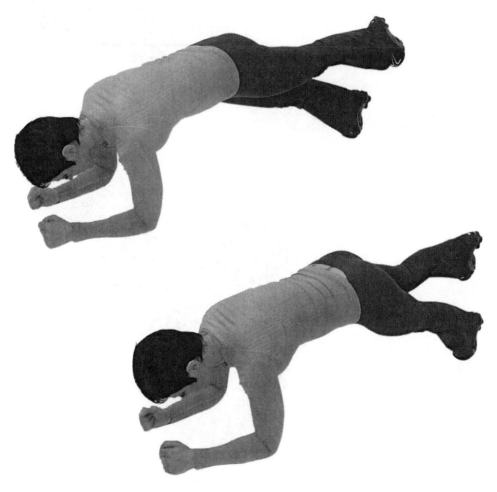

JACK KNIVES

You must pull your upper and lower body up at the exact same time and end with only your butt touching. If you feel this in your back too much, bend your knees a little, and if that doesn't work, your abs may be too weak to do this move right now.

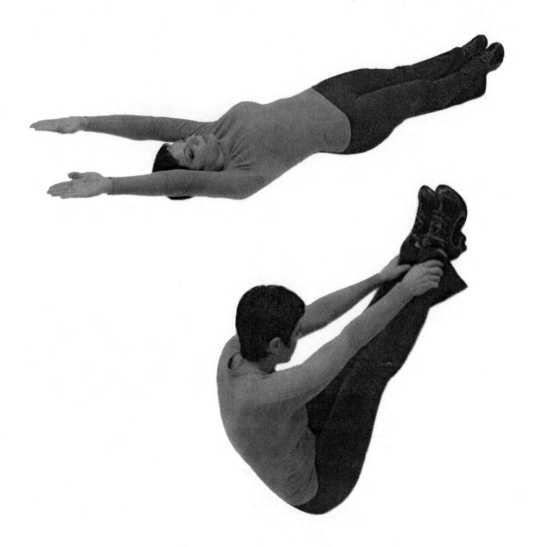

STRADDLE JACK KNIVES

Same as JACK KNIVES, only when you come up, open your legs into a straddle and reach your arms through them. These are a bit easier than JACK KNIVES.

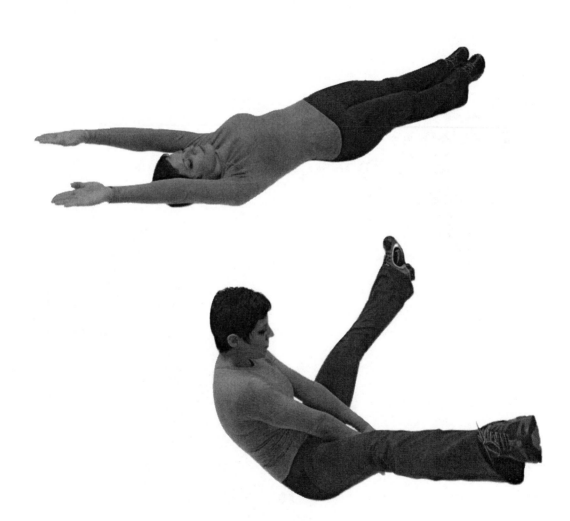

STANDARD SIT-UPS

Just make sure when you come down, you touch your low and midback on the floor, not your shoulders. Touching your shoulders will disengage your abs and make you use your hip flexors attached into your low back.

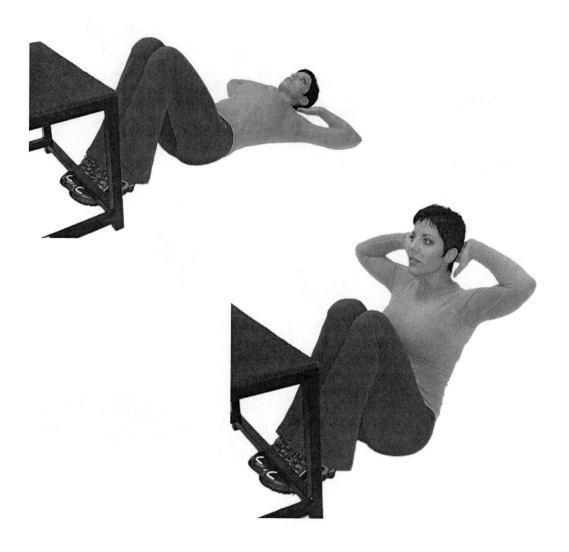

STANDARD SIT-UPS (SIDE TO SIDE)

Same as a SIT-UP only you will twist and touch an elbow to the opposite knee. Come all the way down and then back up to the alternate side. Do not touch the shoulders to the floor once you start.

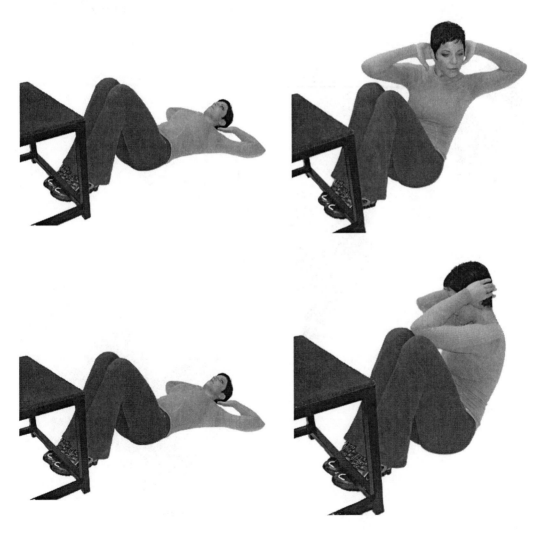

STANDARD SIT-UPS (BOXING TWIST)

When you come up, you will twist and touch an elbow to opposite knee real quick on both knees. Left elbow touches first, then right, then lay back and come up. Now touch right elbow first, then left elbow, quick twist. Keep alternating which elbow you hit first and keep twisting quick at the top.

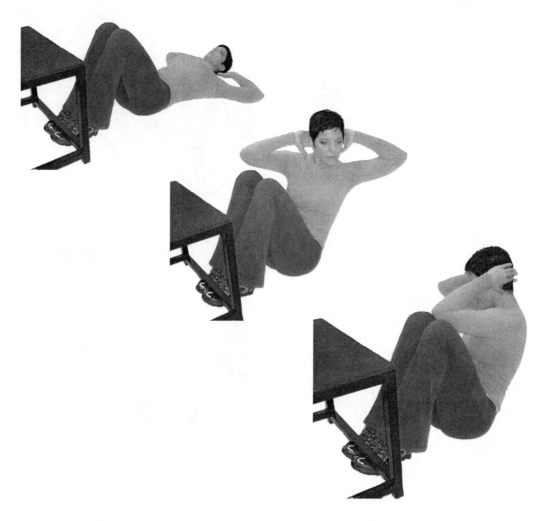

"V" SIT TWIST

Do not arch your back; you need to hunch forward and pull your knees toward your chest. You may use straight arms, reaching out holding a broomstick, or arms bent holding a gallon of water or a weight, touching the floor with the object on each twist. If you have a weak low back, keep your feet on the floor and knees together while you twist.

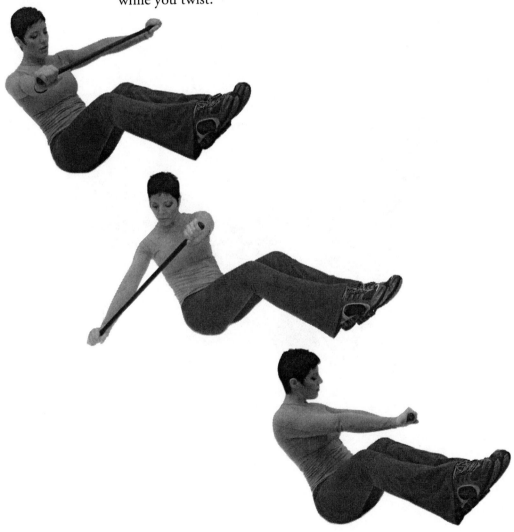

"V" SIT HOLD

Stay hunched forward and your knees pulled close to the chest, palms up to ceiling. The straighter your legs, the harder this exercise becomes.

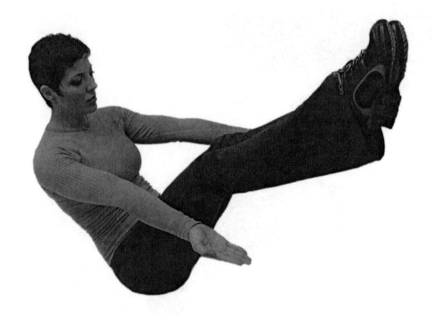

LOW AB CRUNCHES ON THE BALL

To keep the ball from rolling, hold your arms straight and push away as you pull up your legs. Keep a slight bend in your legs and avoid dropping your legs down too far to keep from going into the low back. If you feel it in your back, shorten your "open" range and concentrate on really pulling the knees in. The move mimics the motion of one of those party favors that you blow, they open up, then curl back.

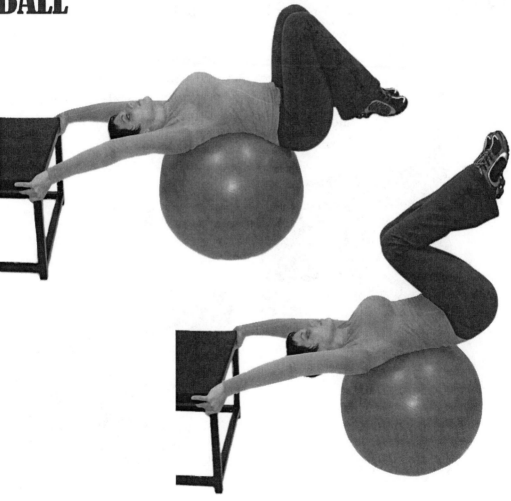

STRAIGHT CRUNCHES ON THE BALL

Any time you do abs on a ball, you get a better range and more out of your crunches. Make sure that you are right on top of the ball so you get the benefit of feeling the negative (opening up). If you have weak abs, you will feel this in your back, so you will need to move the body down more, and do not lay right on top of the ball until you get stronger. Keep your chin up and do not pull on the neck. Most people feel their neck a lot during abs because they have weak neck muscles from looking down too much or at a computer too long. After a couple of weeks, all my clients who complain about their neck during abs, stop complaining because they are stronger, not only in their neck but also in their abs. Lift shoulder only off of the ball and then lightly tap them coming down. It's a very small movement.

SIDE TO SIDE CRUNCHES ON THE BALL

Same as CRUNCHES ON THE BALL only now you will reach to one side, come back, and then reach to the other side. Keep your butt squeezed and thrust your hips to the ceiling during all crunching on the ball. Do not use your legs to help you, and only bring your shoulders up off of the ball, not your midback, that is too far. The correct ab crunches have a very small range to avoid going into your back.

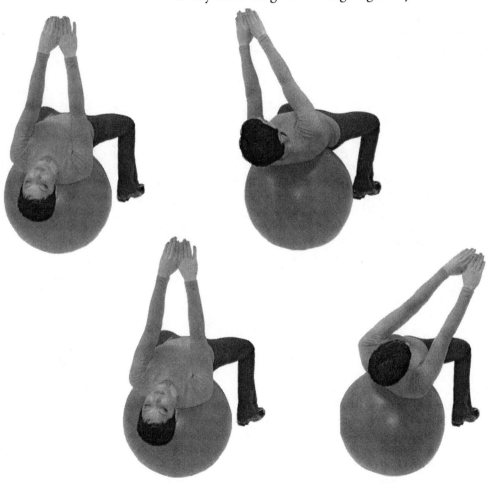

SIDE CRUNCHES ON THE BALL

Your top leg is always in front, keep your hips forward and butt tight. The first reach hits right on the sides of your abs, and the second reach, where you twist with both hands, will really hit your obliques (the side muscles of the abs). Touch your body down to the ball each time and slightly come up, not really high. Avoid using your elbow to push off the ball to help you get up.

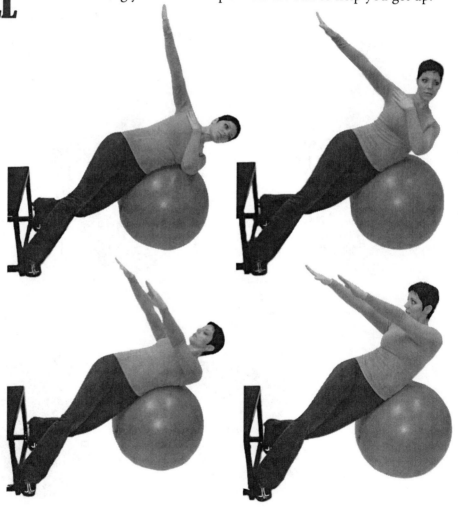

SIDE PLANKS ON ELBOW/ CRUNCHES

Make sure to engage your lats (your back muscles that go from the armpits to the lower spinal area and look like wings when flexed) in the armpit area by pushing away from the floor with the elbow you are on. Do not sink into your shoulder socket. Arch up as high as you can, crunching your side abs. Come down slowly on the negative to avoid having your feet slide away from you. Keep your feet stacked and legs straight.

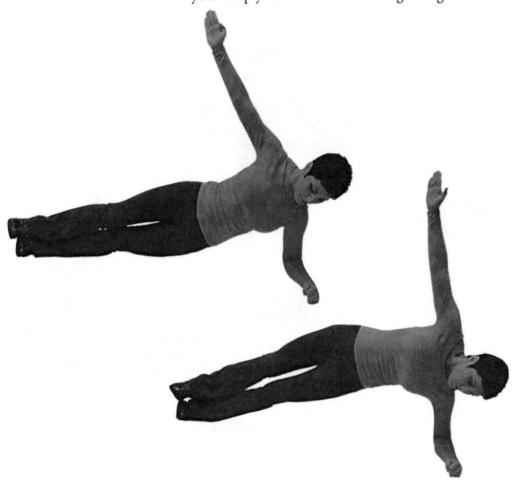

SIDE PLANK HOLD ON HAND

Side plank on hand, making sure to engage your lats by pushing away from the hand you are on. Crunch your side up and lift as high as you can. If you are strong enough, lift your top leg up also and hold.

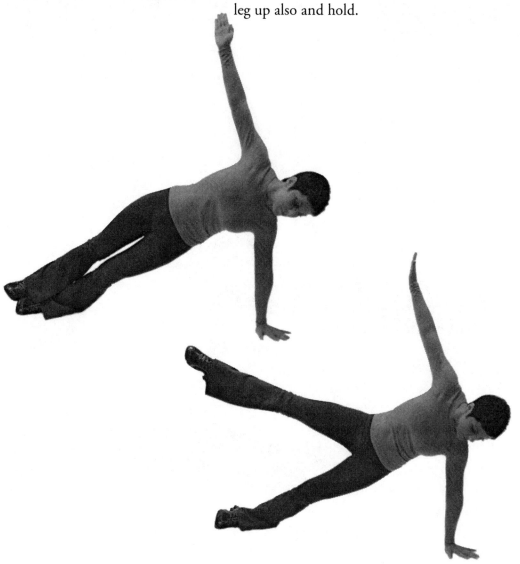

PLANK ON ELBOWS WITH WIDE-LEG STANCE

Keep your bellybutton pulled in and hips tucked under. Keep your legs locked straight and avoid dumping into the low back.

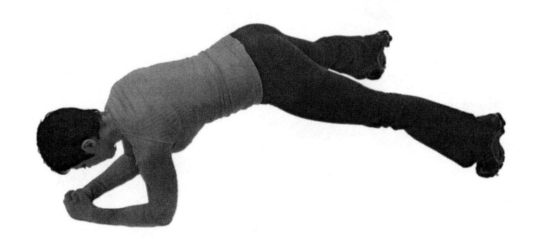

PUSH-UP/ ALTERNATE SUPERMANS

Keep your bellybutton pulled in tight. Squeeze the back of the shoulder blade area of arm and butt muscle of opposite leg and extend out as you come up from the push-up. Go back down into the push-up and extend out the other arm and leg as you come up. Make this move flow as smooth as possible.

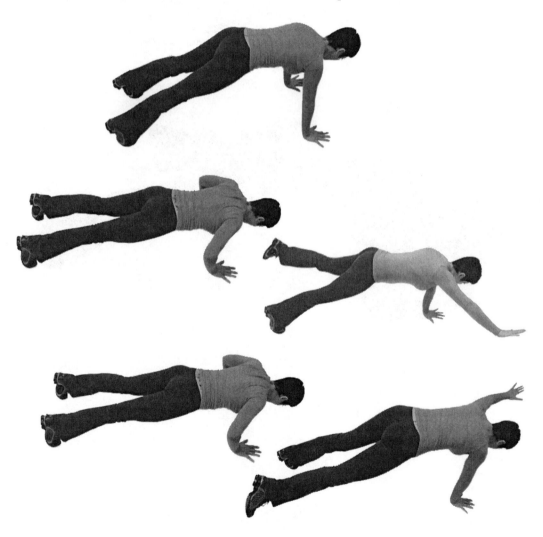

PUSH-UP/ OBLIQUE PULL TO SIDE PLANK

As you come up from the push-up, pull your right knee in to touch the left elbow. As your right foot comes back onto the floor, stack your feet and end up in a side plank on your right arm. Out of the side plank, drop right into a push-up, now pulling your left knee into your right elbow. Once your left foot has gone back and touched the floor, stack your feet and do a side plank on your left arm.

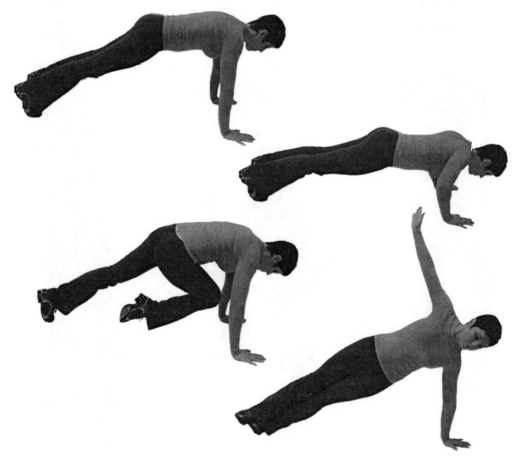

WIDE SQUAT TO A CALF RAISE AND PRESS ABOVE HEAD

Using gallon jugs of water, weights, or a rubber band, wide squat and as you come all the way up into a calf raise (press up on the balls of your feet), also press the weight above the head in one move. Drop everything back down into a deep, wide squat.

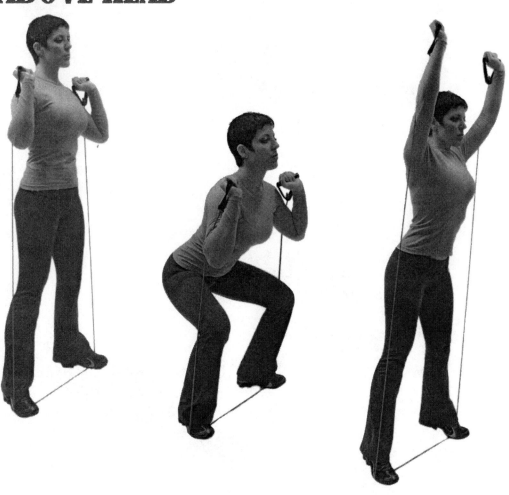

STRAIGHT SQUAT INTO A CALF RAISE PULLING INTO AN UPRIGHT ROW

Wrap a resistance band around the foot of your bed or heavy object. Stand back with feet hip width apart; squat down first. As you stand up, pull up on band into a calf raise, finishing with arms at the top with elbows up high and hands at sternum, doing an upright row. Bring arms down and drop down into straight squat again.

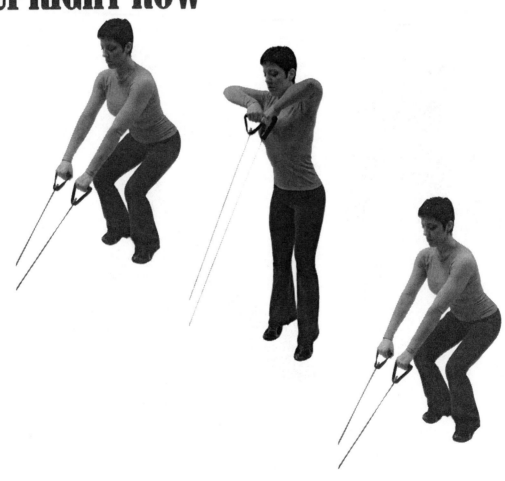

STANDING LUNGE UP INTO LATERAL RAISE AND SIDE KICK

Put a resistance band under your front foot. Go down in a lunge, letting the band relax. As you come up, kick back leg out to the side, as you raise the band into a lateral raise, chest up and abs in. Let the band relax and drop back down into the lunge again. Go up and down smoothly, kicking out to the side and raising elbows.

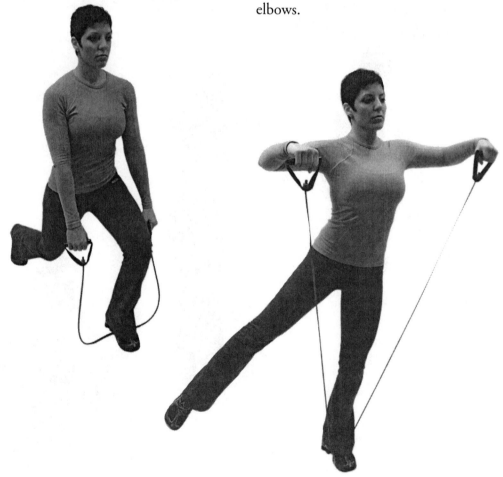

90 DAYS
TO A NEW YOU

PART III

The Detox Program

12 TESTIMONIALS

"Don't compromise yourself. You are all you've got"
—Janis Joplin

THESE ARE SOME TESTIMONIALS FROM SOME OF THE CLIENTS I HAVE WORKED WITH through the years. I asked them to be honest and give advice as if one of their friends or loved ones asked them about doing my three-dimensional program which has become known as The Angela Jordan System.

Donna Mullin: It is with great resolve, that after half a lifetime of trying different diet plans, workout routines, and mantras, I finally figured out the answer to it all. Thanks to A.J., at Camp A.J., the lesson is simple, wise, and strong. When you mentally decide that there are no more excuses, and you want to live a life of health and passion, it can be done. My experience is a familiar one, years of trying new eating habits for a while, years of trying new exercise routines for a while, and years of overall not feeling solid with who I am. Through the recommendation of a friend, I started what I thought was "another try at a temporary solution." To my delight, it has literally changed my life. Through the professional, one-on-one guidance of a well-trained athlete, the guidance of a superb nutritionist, and the psychological healing of many years of self-doubt and unacceptable thoughts, I feel healthier and stronger than ever.

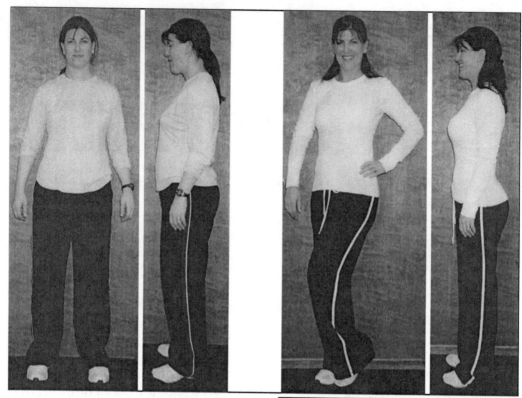

I am not saying that it is easy or magical. In fact, it can be one of the most difficult things you will do.

Let me paint a picture for you. Start with giving up all of your vices: no alcohol, no

Total inches lost: 22 inches!	
Chest- 3 ½	Thigh- 2 ½
Shoulders- 2 ½	Calf- ½
Waist- 6	Bicep- ½
Hips- 5 ½	

Diet Coke™ or coffee, no anything but water in the beginning. You may feel the headache, the irritability, the lack of your "comfort drink," not to mention lack of your "comfort food," which you learn is just a crutch anyway. Food, forget it, it's just for nourishment for a while, and then becomes a lifestyle that actually, really, truly, makes you FEEL better. In the beginning, however, you eat certain proteins, certain carbs, no taste, at first. It's a happy day when you get to add a fruit, and eventually you eat like a normal person again, but decide what is really worth it. I still live for my Diet Cokes. I just learn to drink them with food and limit them in my week. I still have a propensity for sugar and enjoy it tremendously when I make the decision to eat the chocolate cream pie. A.J. will, in fact, notice it on you, in your bloating stomach and your expanding thighs, and she will make you pay for it with very focused exercises on the area that gave it away.

I can say now that not only have I lost many inches, but also I know that my core is strong, vibrant, and capable of many years of an active lifestyle. I am finally okay with the fact that I wear a "large" in skirts. I am an athlete. I will always have to get pants to fit my shape, but that shape isn't so bad, and I am doing my best and feel great! In addition, I wake up knowing exactly what I have to do to be successful and healthy. With no more excuses, I stick to a simple, healthy way of life. I truly enjoy the times when I eat dessert or drink another cocktail, and I don't let it sabotage my plan from there on out. The bull about this being a "way of life" is actually true. You just need the right plan and the right person to take you through it. There are no more excuses.

It is with sincere gratitude for the guidance, the professionalism, the counseling, and the no-nonsense style that I can honestly say thanks to A.J. and Camp A.J. that I have slowly and consistently adopted a healthier and much happier way of life. It positively affects my days, my relationship with my husband and children, and my overall attitude of empowerment. I am forever grateful, and forever making "me" a priority.

Respectfully, Donna Mullin

DONNA WORKED OUT WITH ME ONLY THREE DAYS A WEEK FOR 30 MINUTES. SHE couldn't believe that's all it took physically. This also proved to her that when it comes to your weight, the majority of it has to do with what you put in your mouth.

Ninfa Lowe—I never realized how much sugar I was eating until I talked to Angela. I have tried several diets in the past, and all of them made me go right back to sugar the minute I was off of them.

The problem with most diets is they starve you and drop your calories so low, it's not realistic. I never lost all of my pregnancy weight from my four children who are now all grown up and out of the house.

Trying The Detox was not an easy task, but not because you are starving, that's for sure! You eat all the time on this thing!

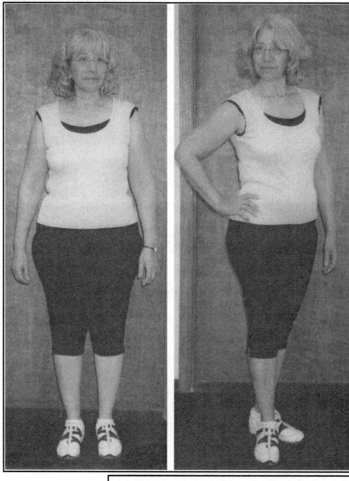

I found what was hard was to be prepared every day with my meals. You never realize how much you don't take care of yourself or pay attention to yourself, until you have to. My family thought it was weird that I had to eat every three hours, but then they eventually supported me and could see that my body was changing, and I had so much more energy during the day. I used to be

Total inches lost: 21 1/2 inches!	
Chest- 3 ½	Thigh- 1 ½
Shoulders- 3	Calf- 1 ½
Waist- 5	Bicep- 2 ½
Hips- 4 ½	

tired around midmorning. I realized I was eating the wrong thing for breakfast.

The Detox makes you eat five balanced meals every day. I never knew how much I snacked on sugar snacks until I replaced them with nutritious meals. I also couldn't believe that my body changed as much as it did with only working out one 30-minute strength training session a week and one 30-minute Pilates™ session a week. I trained for an hour a week, and I lost five inches off my waist! That definitely showed me that the majority of your weight gain and loss has to do with your eating habits.

The Detox really taught me how to eat for life. Now I can always tell when I miss my meals because I feel so low in energy and my body just does not function as well.

Even my children took to the program, and they love it. My daughter is in the fashion retail business. She lost so many inches that her colleagues didn't even recognize her! The Detox is definitely worth your time and effort. You will not be disappointed.

Kris Anderson—I have always done the high protein, no carb thing when I wanted to lose weight. I would eat a lot of chicken and beef with a lot of salads. I would also start running a lot. Once I felt like I dropped enough weight, I would stop running and start to enjoy a sandwich once in awhile, maybe have pizza and a beer on a weekend, and I would just start adding the weight back on faster and more than before. It's like my body couldn't process carbs anymore, but not eating carbs was not realistic for me for a long-term life commitment.

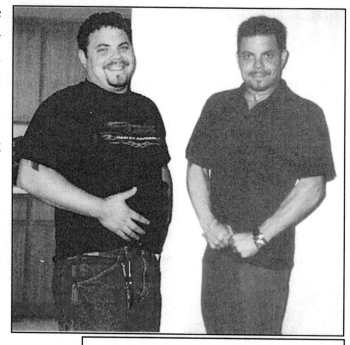

Total lost: 9 inches!
From size 38" waist to 29" wasit.

The Detox was my answer. It's like what I used to do, only I get to eat carbs, too! I could eat oatmeal, rice, and sweet potatoes. I also started more resistance training and not as much running. I lost more body fat weight and had a harder body than when I ate the all protein/no carb diet. I was skinny with that program, but I was soft looking. Angela called it a "skinny-fat." Not the way a man wants to be described. After The Detox, I held more muscle mass, less body fat, and I felt stronger. On the no carbs diet, I always felt low in energy.

Once I finished The Detox, I was able to still go out and enjoy a pizza and some beer or even go for a sandwich for lunch without gaining weight. Sometimes I feel a little bloated from the yeast, but after a day or two, my abs look great! The Detox teaches a way of life, not a fad for the moment. I could never hold the muscle I'm holding now by doing the no carb thing. Carbs are muscle power and body fat burners!

Nancy Anderson—FAT. Yes, there are kinder, gentler words for it, like pleasingly plump, robust, even statuesque. Let's face it, it's FAT! Tired, unhappy, depressed, all because of the FAT!

Like most dieters, I have tried them all. Some worked short-term, some not at all. The Detox is NOT a diet. It's a way of life program! Angela asked me to give her 30 days, just 30 and then I could decide whether to continue or not. I read her Detox program and immediately had the following thoughts:

No caffeine! I can't live without it!

No seasonings! I need them!

No bread! But it's a staple!

No dairy! There go the Dove™ bars!

One gallon of water! I'll need to stay close to a restroom!

Eat every three hours! My schedule is too hectic, there's NO way I can get that many meals in!

With all that said, I decided it was only 30 days out of the rest of my life, I can do this! I discovered Angela's statements

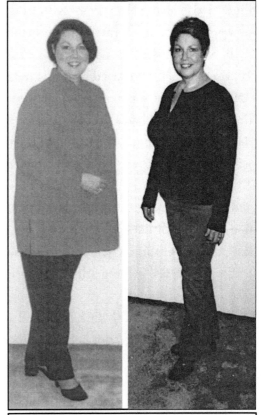

Total inches lost: 33 inches!

Chest- 5 ½	Thigh- 2 ½
Shoulders- 2 ½	Calf- 1
Waist- 10 ½	Bicep- 3 ½
Hips- 7 ½	

about The Detox program were true. It's NOT A DIET, it's a program that helps YOUR body tell you what is making you fat. The key to success is knowledge is power, and this program gives you the power to understand exactly what foods are triggering weight gain. Finally. I can look at certain foods and say to myself, "You can't eat that, your body will not process it correctly and you will gain five pounds of water in no time!" I also learned to stay away from the scale! The only numbers I pay attention to now are my measurements! Muscle weighs more than fat.

In four months I dropped from a size 22 jeans to a size 10! I have never been a size 10! Exercise helps. I started by doing nothing more than walking around the block. At 230 pounds, just walking to the mailbox was exhausting. I started moving better, getting lighter, and I had so much more energy. I started working out three times a week. As the inches dropped, the happier I became. I can walk a flight of stairs without being winded! I can get in and out of a car without grunting! Life is just so much easier!

I followed the first 30-day program to the letter. The second 30 days were heaven and hell. Seasonings were less than half of what I normally used, finding out that my body actually dislikes certain breads, veggies, and fruit was a blessing in disguise! The last 30 days, putting together a maintenance program, was challenging, but so worth it! Losing the fat, gaining self-confidence, and learning how to live longer by living a healthier lifestyle!

This program, NOT DIET, helped me understand my body and how to avoid certain foods that hurt, not help, me. Thanks to AJ's program, I am now eating to live, not living to eat!

Les Anderson: It was the spring of 2003, and I had made a major decision. I was going to throw myself into a new career. This was timed to a major move in our life, leaving Illinois to come to Arizona.

In preparation for these moves, I figured what the heck, I'll go and get a full physical while I have insurance at my employer. The results were not what I had planned for.

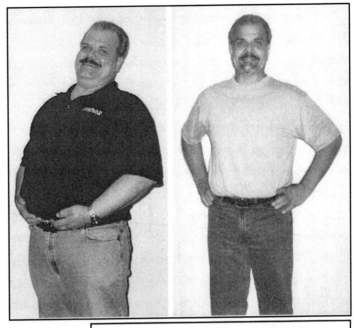

Total inches lost: 16 inches!

From size 54" waist to 38" waist.

I had always been heavy, but I knew that I was bigger than I had ever been. I stayed away from scales because I really didn't want to know.

My doctor told me I was clearly overweight at 346 pounds, I was borderline diabetic, my blood pressure was dangerously high, and my acid reflux had eaten a hole in my throat. Without further discussion, he began writing prescriptions and explaining what my future was going to include.

This is when I said no. No to prescriptions, no to surgical procedures, no to my present lifestyle, and no to accepting the future being planned out by my doctor. My doctor was visibly upset and accused me of giving up. I told him that in my mind following his directions was giving up and that I wanted to know how much of my condition could be changed or controlled. This settled him down but he clearly remained skeptical.

You need to know that at this point I seriously loved life and this lifestyle had taken its toll on my body. I loved work, food (all), drink (all), and fun (all). This left little time for exercise, sleep, and the other things that had seemed less important to me at that time. He almost jokingly told me I would need to lose 100 pounds minimum, eat right, and give up salt, caffeine, and alcohol. He continued to try to persuade me to take blood pressure medicine as well as something for my acid reflux. He also told me he had given this list of things to do to many other patients but had rarely seen the required results. They apparently had found it easier to cut and medicate.

Well, not me. I used The Detox Diet and exercise plan, and when I returned to the doctor, the results were way better that he would have ever expected possible. My blood pressure and sugar levels were well into the norms. My weight was coming down at an amazing rate, and my acid reflux was all but nonexistent, so my throat was healing well. He basically told me that whatever I was doing, just keep doing it.

I really didn't need him to tell me I was doing well, I could *feel* the difference. I now maintain my weight at least 100-120 pounds lighter, and to my delight, I can have all of my favorite foods and drinks in moderation.

I have integrated exercise permanently into my life. I almost never need an antacid and sleep without acid reflux, (I used to need Maalox™ on my bed stand.) By far, the biggest benefit I have received is understanding food, eating, and its effects on my body.

I now do not feel like I am being restricted in any way. I feel like I am making choices that are good for me at any point in time, and I am making choices for the right reasons.

At least once a year I revisit The Detox plan. I always feel better after doing it. I don't believe doctors are bad, but I do think that they take the easiest path: cut and medicate. I will always make these choices my last resort. Thanks to The Detox plan and the help of my daughter, I am now healthier than I was in high school and loving life.

13 GET R.E.A.L. (REALIZE, EVALUATE, ACTION, LIVE)

*"To uncover your true potential,
you must first find your own limits and
then have the courage to blow past them"*
—Picabo Street

Let's do a reality check. Wait! Don't close the book! Now come on! Until you really take a look at yourself and your habits, you will never be able to change. You need to answer each question that follows extremely honestly. No matter how bad it hurts you to realize it. You must "Realize" your emotional and physical issues with food and eating patterns. You must "Evaluate" what you are willing to do and/or not do to reach your goal. Once you have established what you are willing to do, you put it into "Action." By continuing your "Actions," you will now "Live" your new lifestyle. What you have to understand is what's happening on the inside is already showing on the outside. You can't lie to yourself anymore because your health is paying for it.

Turn the page and answer the each of the questions in the space provided:

How long have you been your current size?

_____

_____

What size would you like to be?

_____

How many hours per night do you sleep?

_____

How much water do you drink per day?

_____

How many COMPLETE MEALS do you eat per day?

_____

Checkmark the items below that you consume, then record next to each the portion and how often per day:

Caffeine: _____

Sugar: _____

Red meat: _____

Alcohol: _____

Yeast products: _____

Salty foods: _____

Fatty fried foods: _____

What is your "vice" for the day? (Your comfort food.)

Why do you think you hold weight? (Be brutally honest.)

Do you feel you eat because you are (check all that apply):

Happy

Sad/Depression

Lonely

Bored

Angry/Pissed off

Social Eater

TV Eater

Reward Yourself Eater

Overhungry so you binge eat

What are you not willing to give up to reach your goal?

_____

_____

_____

_____

_____

_____

_____

_____

What time at night are you still putting food into your
mouth?

_____

_____

Do you consume large portions per meal?

_____

How many times per week do you eat out?

_____

How many times per week do you eat fast food?

_____

What's your excuse for missing meals during the day? (Check all that apply.):

_____ No time

_____ Hate cooking

_____ Not hungry

_____ Lazy

_____ Not prepared (No food readily available)

Now let's get even more detailed as to why you eat the way you do.

Write three average days of eating (midweek). Write the time you awaken and the time you go to bed. EVERYTHING you put in your mouth and the time you do it.

Day One:

Day One (Continued):

Day Two:

_____

_____

_____

_____

_____

_____

_____

_____

_____

_____

_____

_____

_____

_____

_____

_____

_____

Day Three:

_____

_____

_____

_____

_____

_____

_____

_____

_____

_____

_____

_____

_____

_____

_____

_____

_____

_____

_____

Now that you have written down your past three days of eating, look for these key elements:

How many COMPLETE MEALS did you eat (containing protein, veggies, and complex carbs)?

How many hours between your meals?

How many hours between awakening and eating?

How many hours between eating and going to bed?

Did you eat complex carbs (rice, potatoes, bread, etc.) in your last meal?

Did you eat protein in every meal?

Did you eat veggies in every meal?

Looking at the portions in each meal, how did each day look? Like an upside down triangle, right side up triangle, or hourglass shape?

How much water did you drink per day?

How much caffeine did you take in per day?

List your simple carbs (bread, pastas, crackers, muffins, etc.):

List your complex carbs (rice, oatmeal, sweet potatoes):

List your condiments (salt, pepper, sauces, dressings):

_____

_____

_____

List what you are doing right:

_____

_____

_____

_____

_____

_____

_____

_____

_____

_____

_____

_____

_____

_____

Now that you have dissected your eating habits, look at your average three days of eating and write down how you feel about what you have discovered.

Now I want you to decide what one thing are you willing to commit to doing that you are not currently doing right now. Think real hard. Search deep inside your soul. Come on. Today, you are moving forward with your health. What one thing will you commit to doing? Maybe it's The Detox. Maybe that is too much for you emotionally. How about a modified Detox? Eat the way you eat for the first 30 days but add the first two weeks of the second 30 days right away. So, basically, you are cutting out dairy and simple carbs (breads, pasta, etc.). You are eating like The Detox in the first 30 days but you are able to have condiments (not drench), and fruit twice per day. Maybe that is also too hard for you emotionally. Maybe you want to commit to just cutting all your portions in half. Maybe you want to commit to eating something every three hours. It doesn't have to be strict.

Make your commitment and write it down. Take what you wrote and put it with your Before picture and put it up on your refrigerator or on your bathroom mirror. That will keep you in check every day as to what your goals are for you and your health.

One more thing and it is not going to be easy. Write down your commitment and give it to someone close to you who will keep you accountable to your goals. It's proven that if you tell someone else your intentions for any goal, you have a better chance of following through with it. Just like in any rehab program, you need someone to call when you feel like you're going to lose control. Everyone needs a sponsor no matter how strong you think you are.

You can do this. You will stick to your goals so make it one that is realistic and get that baby down on paper! If you don't have a plan, you don't have a goal. If you don't have a goal, you don't have a direction. If you don't have a direction, you are standing still. Today, you are taking control of your body, your mind, your emotions, and your health

For support
on your Detox journey,
logon to:

www.NinetyDaysToANewYou.com

14 THE DETOX, AN EXPLANATION

"Nothing is particularly hard if you divide it into small jobs."
–Henry Ford

LET'S DETOX! I KNOW YOU CAN DO THIS! THIS IS NOT A NUTRITION PROGRAM YOU HAVE to stick to forever. It is not easy. It takes a big commitment to stick to. You have to stay focused. You have to want the results so badly that you refuse to let anything or anyone get in your way. Did I say it wasn't easy?

The Detox lasts 90 days or three months, whichever sounds better to you. Wait! Don't put the book down yet! Each month is a different process. The first 30 days is your toughest, but I promise, if you can stick to this, you will not be disappointed! I have had clients lose 18 inches or more in one month! I have had clients lose 7-8 inches in two weeks! Please, read on. I know you can do this! The reason I call this a Detox, is because I'm stripping your body of caffeine, sugars, alcohol, yeast, and all condiments. In the second 30 days, I will add in something each week, to see if your body has a reaction to it. An example of a reaction would be gas, bloating, headache, fatigue, hyperness, or stuffy sinuses. Once you see how you react to foods, like bloat when you eat dairy, you know you should limit your consumption of that food to avoid weight gain. The best way to describe a food reaction is, when you go to dinner and even if you don't eat a lot or you don't eat that unhealthy, you can't wait to get to your car so

165

you can unbutton your pants. This means you had a food reaction.

You can't get fat over one meal. Let me say that again. You can't get fat over one meal. Your meal probably had too much sodium or too much dairy or yeast. It's like trying a new lotion on your skin and breaking out in a rash. The Detox will help you see what your body reacts

my clients will redo the first, hard 30-day Detox for only two weeks every time they splurge on a long vacation or after the holidays. It gets your body right back on track, especially since it's already been through the whole thing once before. So are you ready to do this? I know you are.

The first 30 days are the toughest. Once you see those results, you'll fly

...if it didn't work and you SWEAR you did it EXACTLY the way I tell you, then I need you to do a blood test.

to which, over time, will put weight on you. Once you do The Detox, you never have to do it again because you will know what's putting weight on you, if you ever start gaining again. The only job you have is limiting these foods. Start eating too much of that particular food again, and hello weight gain. The third 30 days is putting it all together: Your life plan and way of eating that is sensible for your lifestyle, basically "a way of life" for your eating habits. Remember what I said before, "You are what you eat." Most of

through the next two months to finish the 90-day program. I will mentally and emotionally help you as much as possible to get you through these next four weeks of your life. Be strong, get focused, and let's do this!

The Detox works for everyone! Every one of my clients who has done this and stuck to it exactly was amazed! I tell everyone if it didn't work and you SWEAR you did it EXACTLY the way I tell you, then I need you to do a blood test. You need to check your thyroid and check for diabetes. Those are mainly in charge of your metabolism. But, like I said, The Detox has worked for everyone, including my clients who had thyroid problems or type 2 diabetes. You will see that each meal in The Detox has a protein, a complex starchy carb, a complex fibrous carb, and a good fat. The only meal that has no complex starchy carb is your last one before you go to bed. Remember, eat for your next activity. Going to sleep does not require starchy carbs.

As you look at The Detox, you will notice it is very plain and boring. You are very observant. For the next four weeks, you will be eating for a different reason than you normally do. You are going to "eat to live," not "live to eat." Now I know what you are thinking. "There is no way!" Oh, yes, there is.

For once in your life, get this eating thing figured out!

It is four weeks to focus on your eating habits, your needs, your struggles, and your weaknesses. Come on, I know you can do this! For once in your life, get this eating thing figured out! Now let's take a look at the big, bad Detox. I'm going to explain what you're eating and why. I will tell you what to expect physically, mentally, and emotionally. I want you to be successful. Are you with me? Of course you are, because you're more than ready to change your health and take care of your body. Now take my hand and let's jump in that pool!

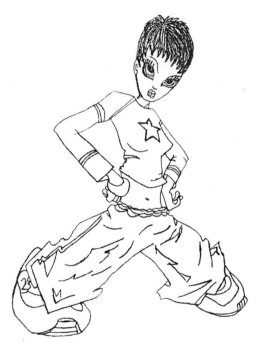

"Focus on one day at a time... get your meals in!"

MEAL 1:

1 whole egg, 1 egg white (2 eggs total) cooked in a quarter-size measure of olive oil

¼-1 cup of cooked cream of rice or oatmeal with a soupspoon-size measure of ground flax seed

MEAL 2:

Protein (size of deck of cards)

¼-1 cup of cooked Uncle Bens™ converted rice, basmati rice, baseball-size yam or sweet potato, brown rice, quinoa, Rice Select Royal Blend™ (texmati white, brown, wild, and red rice)

1 cup of veggies with quarter-size measure of olive oil drizzled on them

MEAL 3:

(Same as meal two)

MEAL 4:

(Same as meal two and three)

MEAL 5:

Protein (size of deck of cards)
2 cups of veggies with quarter-size measure of olive oil drizzled on them

TIPS:

- Eat every three hours

- Drink up to a gallon of water a day

- Do not eat: caffeine, sugar, alcohol, condiments (no salt, pepper, dressings), fruit, dairy

- You may use real spices to spice up food (garlic cloves, onion, peppers, mushrooms, tomatoes)

- Proteins: eggs, chicken, turkey, fish, beef

- Veggies: (no carrots or corn) mostly green veggies

- Bob's Red Mill™ ground flax seed

- Portions can be raised or lowered according to your athletic needs.

- To replace tea or coffee: 1 cup of hot water with a half lemon

If it is not listed here, it does not go into your mouth!

Now are you done whining and complaining about what you can't have? I'm going to explain to you in a little more detail why certain things are on The Detox.

The cup of hot water with a half lemon is used to stimulate and clean the kidneys. Lemon acts as a natural diuretic, helping you to lose water retention. You may cut up lemons and put them in your water all day. You'll find you will pee a lot more, which means you system is cleaning out. It also helps fill the void for the tea or coffee you used to drink, but will not be drinking during the first 30 days. Oh, stop with the face. You can do this.

The portions I have put down in each meal are an average. I have found that some of my female clients do ¼ cup of starchy carbs, whereas my male clients do anywhere from ½–1 cup. Males also tend to have three egg whites with one whole egg, giving them four eggs instead of two. The majority of people do The Detox as you see it.

As far as the one whole egg, you need the good fat from the yolk, since the only other type of fat you will be getting is in the olive oil. I've had clients who don't eat eggs, so they usually have some chicken or a turkey burger for breakfast.

If you don't like oatmeal or cream of rice, use the Uncle Ben's™ converted rice or basmati rice in the morning with your choice of protein. The reason I have you eat cream of rice instead of cream of wheat is because I have found that wheat products tend to make estrogen levels go up, causing water retention. I tend to stay away from wheat products. They can even make males hold fluid in the midsection. I use rice products, quinoa, and gluten-free flours.

The Bob's Red Mill™ ground flax seed is also for the good fats you need. It helps regulate hormone levels in men and women and it helps you stay regular. Yes, going number two.

You can not eat corn or carrots. Corn does not digest and carrots are mostly sugar, which I'm trying to clean out of your system. I know, I know, "But these are the only ones I like," right? Get over it! Eat your greens!

The olive oil you drizzle on them gives them a little flavor. If you do not like cooked veggies you may do a spinach or romaine lettuce salad with lemon squeezed over it. Remember, no condiments; this means no salad dressing. Oh, quit with the faces! You're like a little kid whose mother is trying to get them to eat their vegetables. See, I told you your emotional crud would come out during this. And no condiments. This includes no salt or pepper (there you go again with the face), you may use lemon, olive oil, to it and eat it up as is. No milk, brown sugar, blah, blah, blah. You're going to get wrinkles if you keep making that face. If you can't gag down the plain oatmeal or cream of rice, eat scrambled eggs on top of the converted rice. It's like eating Chinese fried rice. (Sort of. Well maybe not quite that good.) If you absolutely

If you don't eat breakfast you will never be able to stabilize your blood sugar no matter what you eat the rest of the day.

onions, fresh garlic cloves, fresh herbs (none from jars), any kind of fresh peppers (red, green, yellow, hot, mild), and even tomatoes to spice up your food. You may use a homemade salsa only, none of the commercial brands.

Your veggies can be fresh or frozen, no canned. You cannot do egg substitutes instead of the eggs. I prefer you do the slow-cooked oats over the instant, but I do understand people and their time issues. You may do the plain packets of oatmeal, no flavored. You will cook it in water and add your ground flaxseed

NEED to have something in your oatmeal, you may sprinkle a little cinnamon in it. If the ground flax meal makes it too thick, you may put the flax meal in one of your other meals, such as putting it on your rice or mashed sweet potatoes.

The hot water with lemon can be done while you are getting ready in the morning, reading the paper, as an afternoon teatime, and/or relaxing at night in front of the TV.

You will want to vary your proteins. You can have red meat twice per week and salmon three times per week. Everything else, have as many times as you want. Depending on how athletic you are, you may need more red meat because of the natural creatine in the meat to help your muscles recover.

So how are you feeling? The key to the success or failure of this Detox and for the future of your nutrition program is preparation, preparation, and preparation. I cannot say that enough. If you don't have your next meal handy, you are screwed. You will either miss the meal or eat something you shouldn't eat.

I absolutely hate to cook. I cook Saturday night and sometimes on Wednesday nights. You will learn to cook in bulk. Grill 8–10 chicken breasts on the grill along with some veggie shish ka-bobs. You can even bake some sweet potatoes on the grill. I love using my wok. It's fast and simple. I use an easy rice steamer and I steam enough rice for the whole week. The only meal I cook every day is my breakfast. I cook it the night before so all I have to do is throw it in the microwave in the morning.

Remember, I get up at 3 a.m. People who say they've never been breakfast eaters are usually late-night eaters, and that's why they are not hungry in the morning.

Every person who has ever said that has ended up loving breakfast once I took his or her late-night eating away.

You have to remember that if you don't eat breakfast you will never be able to stabilize your blood sugar no matter what you eat the rest of the day. Even if you never do any of my tips in this book again, please keep eating breakfast. You won't believe the effect it will have on your body in the long run.

So, as I was saying, the key to a successful Detox or any nutrition program is preparation, preparation, and preparation! The majority of my clients say this is what made them fail in the first or second week of The Detox. One of my clients started, stopped, and started again six times before they finally got the preparation process down. Just think of it as making your own little TV dinners. You can make several meals, freeze them, and voila, you just have to heat them up!

The more meals you take in, the less your body wants to hold of each one.

As you can see, the only thing you can drink on the first 30 days of The Detox is water. You want to try to get as close to a gallon a day as you can. The more water your body gets, the less water it wants to retain. Just like your meals. The more meals you take in, the less your body wants to hold of each one. You may add lemons to your water to give it a little flavor. No coffee, not even decaf. No teas, not even green tea. Water, that's it. I never said this was fun.

I'm sure you noticed I have five meals in The Detox. As I said earlier, that is not set in stone. If your sleep schedule is off, you may only get in three meals that day. Try your hardest to get no less than three meals a day, and if you have a longer work day, like I do, you may get 6-7 meals in on that day.

Just remember, your last meal has no starchy carbs. The kitchen is closed once you have eaten your last meal! Nothing except water, I mean not even a little something!

There is one more thing you must do before you do The Detox. Take Before pictures (see Testimonials) and measurements. You can do weight also. I always stick to measurements because your weight is more if you hold a lot of muscle mass. No one can ever guess my weight. Besides, the inches are what show. You don't wear your weight number on your forehead for everyone to see. Most of my clients hate when I do Before pictures and measurements, but once they finish the 90 days, they love the After pictures when compared with the Before pictures. Plus, the Before picture reminds them of where they don't want to end up again. So smile pretty!

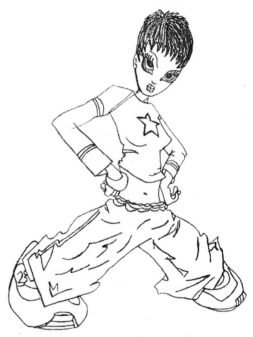

"Focus on what you're supposed to eat... not what you can't eat!"

15 THE CONTRACT

"It is our duty to proceed as if limits to our abilities do not exist."
—Pierre Teilhard de Chardin

ACKNOWLEDGE IT · FACE IT · LOSE IT FOR GOOD · THEN LIVE IT

I HAVE PUT TOGETHER THIS CONTRACT SO YOU CAN PUT YOUR COMMITMENT TO YOUR weight loss program in writing. When you put your intentions and goals on paper in black and white, it makes it all become very real! It's easy to think to yourself, "I'll start eating better on Monday." Then Monday comes and goes. How many times have you done this before? You will also notice on my contract that you have to have one other person be responsible for motivating you to your goal. This makes you accountable! This makes it become very real! Now you have someone else who also knows your intentions and goals and has made it their priority to do everything they can to motivate you and help you accomplish your goal. Pick this person wisely! This is like when a person in AA has a sponsor to check in with or call if they feel they need support. It is easy to THINK about starting a weight loss program. It is a total different story when you tell someone, sign something, and involve that person on your journey to health!

I _____ will participate in

90-Day Detox

14-Day Detox

Getting rid of one bad food for 14 days (name the food)

I _____ will support _____

in his/her commitment by checking in every day to help him/her stick to the program and complete his/her goal. I _____ will be available for _____ to call me anytime he/she needs my support.

I _____ will be strong and stay focused on my goal and allow my supporter _____ to step in and help me whenever I'm in need of extra strength. I will do the following acts to accomplish my goal: _____

_____

Upon accomplishing my goal of _____

_____ ,

I will _____ , and then continue to take on this new way of life, even after reaching my goal, to protect my health and body and to be here for all my friends and loved ones because I am very special in this world and everyone needs me to be here for a long time. I have things to give and things to offer, and by taking care of my health, I will be able to accomplish those things.

DATE:

BOTH SIGNATURES

_____

_____

Make sure to list everything you will do, as in physically, to accomplish your goal. Be very precise with your information. Also, be very precise with listing your goal, and with listing what you will do after you accomplish your goal. Maybe you'll go shopping for new clothes, maybe take a beach vacation, or maybe you'll buy yourself a special gift to mark the moment. Just make sure to be very precise in your contract because that makes it REAL.

The other person who signs this contract needs to take it seriously and must understand how important it is to you to reach this goal. This is your supporter to whom you will go to when you need help, so choose wisely.

This contract needs to be on your refrigerator or on your bathroom mirror at all times. It needs to be visible where you will see it every day. Make more copies and put them up in every room if you need to.

If you do not reach your goal at the time you have chosen, you must redo another contract. You must figure out why the first goal wasn't reached. Do you need to change your goal? Do you need to change your actions to get to that goal?

Do you need a new supporter? Do not do the same contract twice! Take this seriously and you will succeed. Remember:

"If you don't have a goal,

Then you don't have a plan.

If you don't have a plan,

Then you don't have

A direction.

If you don't have a direction,

Then you're sitting still!"

Get a goal,

Make a plan.

Have some direction,

And get somewhere!

16 DETOX BLUES

"You've got to get up every morning with determination
if you're going to go to bed with satisfaction."
–George Lorimer

HERE ARE SOME MENTAL, EMOTIONAL, AND PHYSICAL THINGS YOU CAN EXPECT WHILE on The Detox.

WEEK 1: Extreme fatigue, extreme moodiness, may feel bloated or have gas, joint and/or body aches, extreme caffeine headaches, possibly have to stay in bed and miss work, you may vomit from the headaches, insulin lows, no strength in the gym, wanting to give up, obsessed with what you can't eat or drink, irregular pooping schedule or constipation, unbelievable cravings.

I'm sure you are looking at these symptoms and saying, "I don't want to feel like this!" Well, let me tell you. The reason you will feel like this is because of the crap you've been putting into your body. Just wait until you reach the end of those 30 days and how much better you are going to look and feel. You will see how much all that caffeine and sugar and sodium were affecting your body. How the alcohol was bloating you and even keeping you from having a restful sleep. My clients going through menopause even noticed better sleep and no more hot flashes! So I think you can see by the above symptoms that your first week on The Detox will be hell. I'm not going to lie. This first week is the hardest one to get through. The weekend is your first big test. Many of my clients cheated on that first weekend and had to start over on Monday. The reason is, you are not on a normal schedule. You may not work or you may have company, or may have parties to go to. There is a lot of temptation on the weekends.

There are many ways to be successful. If you go out to eat, do not look at a menu. You already know what you want. Water with lemon, a dry salad with lemon—no cheese, no croutons, no fruit and no seasonings. For a meal, a plain grilled piece of fish or a small fillet and plain steamed veggies. If you go for sushi for dinner, you can't eat the rice. If you go to a party, eat your meal before you go.

All of my clients who make it past that first weekend always make it through the next three weeks. Most of my clients try to schedule this Detox when they don't have as many functions to go to, or trips or other temptations that make The Detox even harder.

WEEK 2: Still some fatigue, weakness in the gym, headaches should be letting up, sleeping more soundly and heavily, still moody (especially if you are an emotional eater), feeling less bloated and your stomach may even seem flatter, your face may even start to look thinner.

You're in week two!! Congrats to you! Week two is not as bad, but still a challenge. Some people still feel tired during the day and even winded when they try to do any physical activities. This is your body still wanting to rely on caffeine and sugar for energy. It hasn't quite started attacking your fat cells just yet. Your body still thinks you're joking with all this nonsense and you're going to have that cup of coffee or cookie soon! Emotionally, I have clients go either way at the end of week two.

Most clients feel like they are over the hump and only have two weeks to go. Plus, they can tell by how their clothes fit that they have already lost some inches. Now I do have that handful of clients who say after two weeks, "I quit." Even after I pull out the tape measure and show them they have lost 6-8 inches all over! Emotionally, they are defeated, and it's not worth it to them to continue. One thing they do realize when they take that weekend at the end of week two and splurge, they physically pay for it. They decide to eat everything and drink everything, all at once, in a matter of two days. Amazing how powerful the emotions are! After eating like this, they realize how bad their body feels when it has that sugar, caffeine, and alcohol back in it. Every single one of my clients who has done this quit-and-splurge phase, has gone back on The Detox and successfully completed it.

Your mind and your emotions can have extreme powers over your physical being. No matter what nutrition program or new diet you want to try, your mind and emotions are just not ready to let go yet. I say it's time you take the power back, and you reclaim the body and the health you deserve.

WEEK 3: More energy and stamina, strength in the gym, emotionally more stable, becoming more regular with the bathroom, amazingly deep, restful sleep, amazing mental focus and calmness during the day, younger, clearer skin, body shape changing in losing inches and weight.

You're in week three! You're half-way there! Stay focused! All my clients are amazed at how good they feel, even though they are eating the same thing as the last two weeks. In week three the body gives in and says, "Fine, don't give me all the crap food, caffeine, and sugar." The body finally decides, "I'll just pull from your fat cells for energy." YES! That's what I'm talking about! This is the process you've been waiting for. Your own body goes after its own body fat. You do realize that you're probably eating double what you were eating before and losing weight on it. See, we got that fire in your belly burning strong! Your metabolism is flying! This is the week a lot of my clients have people mention they are noticing some changes in their body.

WEEK 4: Lots of energy, great looking skin, loss of inches and weight, amazing sleep, excellent mental focus, positive attitude, fewer body aches.

It's week four! You're on the home-stretch! You are so going to finish this Detox! Believe it or not, a lot of my clients almost feel sad that they are in the final week of the hard part. They feel such a sense of accomplishment and their body is functioning so well, they don't want to do anything to screw it up. Your body is functioning like a fine-tuned machine by the end of week four. You're in a groove.

Making it to this point without one cheat is a major accomplishment! You should be very proud of yourself. My clients tell me they can't believe how much better they feel without all the sugar, caffeine, and alcohol in their body. They love how much energy they have all day because of getting all their meals in every three hours. They also have a better understanding of their emotions and reasons for eating the way they did before The Detox.

In week four, you may reflect back to how awful you felt in week one. It can make you realize how much extra "stuff" you were putting in your body that was hurting you physically, but satisfying you mentally and emotionally. Most of my clients will tell me, "I never want to feel like that again." They are shocked when I say to them, "You will, but only at certain times." Those times would be: holidays, vacations, birthdays, weddings, celebrations, or trying new foods. I mean, come on. Nobody is perfect. Remember what I said in the beginning. The Detox is used to clean your system out the first 30

days. The second 30 days is to reintroduce foods back into the body each week to see how the body reacts. The third 30 days is to figure out a maintenance program or, as I call it, "a way of life." One of my top Detox winners told another one of my clients, "You have to change your relationship with food." I thought that was awesome that she got that from doing the 90-day Detox challenge at my gym.

Once you have finished week four, remember to take new measurements. You can take new pictures, also. I usually always take the final picture at the end of the 90 days. That way, you have a Before and an After. Measurements and weight you do every 30 days. You should be so proud of what you have just accomplished! You have also had your last week of bland food! Now let's add some flavor!

On the following pages, write what emotions came up for you during the first 30 days. What physical effects did you feel?

17 DON'T EVEN THINK ABOUT QUITTING

"Consistency and persistence will get you to your goal."
–Unknown

Flavor!

YOU HAVE MADE IT TO THE SECOND 30 DAYS! YOU FINALLY GET FLAVOR! THE GOAL FOR this month is to see how your body reacts once you start putting certain things back into your body. You are still going to eat the same menu as the first 30 days. What!? Yes, you heard me. Your menu is the same as the first 30 days, except for each week you will be adding something more into your program. During these next 30 days, you will be watching to see if you have highs and/or lows in energy after you eat. Watch for bloating or gas. Watch for headaches or stuffed up sinuses. Watch for puffiness under the eyes, or your jewelry fitting tighter. All of these symptoms are signs of your body having a reaction to what you just ate. These are not good things to have. Here's the next 30 days. Enjoy!

WEEK 1: You get condiments back! Very little, do not drench the food. Dip your fork in the sauce and then stab the food, instead of drenching the whole plate.

EXAMPLES: Cinnamon on your oatmeal (cinnamon is a natural blood sugar stabilizer) or light soy sauce on your chicken and rice and veggies.

WEEK 2: You get two pieces of fruit a day! Always eat fruit in your breakfast meal and meal three or four. You can also eat it after your workout.

EXAMPLES: Berries in your oatmeal and an apple with meal three or four. (You may leave condiments in once you have started them in week one.)

WEEK 3: You can have dairy twice a day. Yogurt and cottage cheese are different from milk and yellow cheese. Do them on separate days to see what you have problems with. Milk, ice cream, and yellow cheese make people have bloating because of lactose intolerance. Yogurt and cottage cheese are not processed the same. (No fruit in this week.)

EXAMPLES: Yogurt with your breakfast meal, cottage cheese with meal five; OR milk in your oatmeal and three dice-size pieces of yellow cheese in meal five.

WEEK 4: You get bread and pasta and other yeast or wheat products. Sourdough bread is the best bread for your insulin. Even better than wheat bread. Yep. That's right. It's processed differently that's why it's called SOURdough. (No dairy or fruit this week.)

EXAMPLES: Toast with your eggs in your first meal instead of oatmeal, and pasta with your chicken or beef and veggies in meal three.

Now let me explain these 30 days a little better, and try to answer any questions you might have now that you've read the above plan. Week one is the condiments week. You may use salt, pepper, salad dressings, sauces, etc. Most people will not have too much of a reaction to condiments, but some of you will.

I notice some people get puffy under the eyes or in the jaw line area. They also have some sinus stuffiness, especially if they eat cream sauces or dressings. Most of my clients are surprised at how small an amount of condiments they use on their meal compared to what they used to put on their food. Your taste buds are very sensitive because of not having any condiments for a month. I have cleansed your palate. One of my clients laughed when I said cinnamon is sweet. They used real sugar on everything. Once they did The Detox, they could never go back to sugar again, and they think cinnamon is sweet enough.

I allow condiments to stay in the rest of the month, since they don't affect the body as much as some of the other foods. The main thing to remember is: Do not go back to drenching your food!

You may also have one cup of black coffee or tea. Yes! Caffeine! No creams or dairy until week three. You may use a little sugar. Real sugar is different from the commercial sweeteners. Try one and see how you react and try the other the next morning and see how you react. I prefer that people use the real thing and just limit the portion.

The second week is fruit. Fruit is sugar; even though it is a natural sugar, it is still a sugar. Dried fruit has the highest sugar. Bananas have a lot of sugar, especially the browner the peel is. That is why the best banana bread is made with very brown bananas. They are pure sugar. Apples have great fiber. Remember, an apple a day keeps the doctor away! Berries have great antioxidants which help rid the body of free radicals, which you get from burnt food or the grill marks on food. Most clients will notice some highs in energy and then a very low in energy after eating fruit.

One of my clients had a fruit smoothie made with fruit and protein powder and water. She noticed a rush of energy and then in 20 minutes she wanted to take a nap. I told her she needed to eat an animal protein with the fruit because her body breaks down the fruit and utilizes it quickly. The protein slows that process down. She had a hardboiled egg next time with the smoothie and it helped maintain her energy for up to an hour and a half.

The dairy week is rough on everyone. Most of my clients get bloated and have gas during the dairy week. They also start having sinus trouble and mucus buildup in their throat. I rarely do any dairy. I will do it once in awhile in the form of a cheat called ice cream and I pay dearly for it. My family laughs at how after two bites I sound like I have the worst sinus cold. I can eat yogurt and cottage cheese without having that reaction. I just choose not to eat them very often. I use goat cheese or tofu cheese on my omelet in the morning.

In the last week, most of my clients also know that they will probably bloat when they eat bread and pasta. I tell them they still need to do it so they can see for themselves. That is what this month is for. You really need to concentrate on your body and get to know it for once in your life. It will tell you exactly how it feels about what you are putting in it. You will notice that the piece of wheat toast with your eggs will not sustain your hunger issues as long as the oatmeal you were eating. Oatmeal will last you almost up to the three hours you need. The toast will last maybe an hour and a half, same as the pasta.

As far as portion size of pasta, the amount is the size of the palm of your hand. Yes, that's it. Bread and pasta are simple carbs, remember? Rice and oatmeal and sweet potatoes are complex carbs. Simple carbs leave quickly, complex lasts longer.

At the end of the second 30 days you should have learned a lot about your body. For once in your life, you should finally know what puts weight on you and what makes you have low energy.

One of my clients had this tickle in his throat, a mucus feeling he could never get rid of. It was gone at the end of the first 30 days. He added a dab of cream to his coffee in week three and it came back

by the end of the first day he had that first cup. He couldn't believe it! Know your body. Only you can know it best!

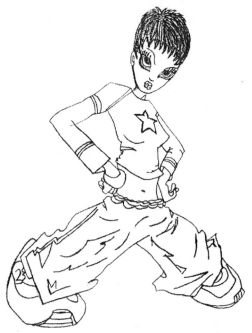

"Your body reacts when it doesn't like what you feed it... LISTEN!"

On the following pages, write what you have learned about your body. What effects and/or reactions did you experience.?

ANGELA JORDAN'S 90 DAYS TO A NEW YOU

18. THE FINAL COUNTDOWN

"To accomplish great things,
we must not only act, but also dream;
not only plan, but also believe."
—Anatole France

YOU HAVE MADE IT TO THE FINAL 30 DAYS! YOU HAD BETTER BE PRETTY PROUD OF yourself right now! What you have done so far has taken so much dedication, will power, and pure focus to get you to your current state of mind and physical being. These last 30 days are used for you to have a real heart-to-heart talk with yourself and ask yourself what you have learned in the last 60 days. This is the month where you put together a life plan for your eating program. Think about all the mental, emotional, and physical stuff you went through in the first 30 days while you were trying to clean out your system. Write it down. It helps to have it look at it and have it staring right back at you. Now think about what your body went through in the second 30 days when you reintroduced into your body some of these foods you used to eat. Be honest with yourself and your body. Once you have written all of this down, take a good look at it and ask yourself how you want your body to feel, to function, to live? What type of program is realistic for you to stick to on a daily basis? What are you willing to give up, what are you not willing to give up when it comes to your favorite foods. I have had clients say, "I don't care if I had painful gas all night from eating cheese, I want it!" I tell them not to eat it every day, and to limit their portions to three cubes the size of dice per meal. As you see, I said per meal. You must eat it with a meal, not alone or with only crackers. The reason is, protein and veggies and complex carbs will help break it down.

I also told my client, "If you start to notice that little pouch coming back in your belly, cut back on the cheese." She knew I was right. I had a client who wanted to put back her one Diet Coke™. I said, that's fine but it has to be with a meal, not alone. She said she had never done that before. She noticed when she did that she was not as bloated after drinking it.

When you go to a restaurant and order your favorite meal, take a good look at it before you start to wolf it down. Ask these questions:

- What is my protein? How is the portion?

- What is my carbohydrate? Is it simple or complex? How is the portion?

- What is my fibrous carb? How is the portion?

- Check out the condiments? Taste it before salting. Heavy sauces?

- Is the overall meal portion too much? Should you take half of it home?

These are some of the questions you should be asking yourself to keep yourself in check with what is going into your body. Some helpful tips for going out, if you want to be on the healthy side, are:

- Ask for condiments on the side

- Ask for steamed veggies instead of sautéed

- Share an entrée with someone or order an appetizer as a meal for portion control

- If you have wine with dinner, skip dessert, or share a small dessert to limit your sugar intake. (Yes, you may have one alcoholic drink per week now.)

In my next chapter I will give you other ways of losing weight or maintaining a good weight for your body. These last 30 days you are to eat just like the first 30 days but add in some of the foods you added in during the second 30 days. You are still getting in 4–5 complete meals. You have flavor, fruit, maybe a little dairy, and on some days you have some toast or a little pasta. You are not to go back to the crazy way of eating you did before The Detox. Why would you want to waste all that time and energy?

Measure yourself for your final measurements at the end of the last week of this last 30 days. Weigh yourself if you are also keeping track of that, and remember to take your final After pictures. Make sure to wear the same outfit you had on in the Before pictures. I always frame the Before and After picture side by side for my clients to have at home so they can remember the transformation of their body. That Before picture also reminds you to never do that to yourself again. You deserve better.

The worst thing you could do to yourself after you have completed The 90-Day Detox is to go back to eating only one or two meals a day again. Even if you add some of your chocolate or your Diet Coke™ or your cheese back in, that won't do near the damage to your body that stopping your meals will do. Why? Remember what I said about the fire burning in your belly. You need food coming in every three hours to keep that fire burning. Do not shut your metabolism down again! Keep your body burning! I had clients tell me that they went to a huge Mexican dinner one night so they only ate their first meal, knowing that they were going to eat and drink a ton at dinner. I told them that was the worst thing they could have done. You need to keep your system on a schedule of every three hours.

Remember what I said, "Every meal you miss, your body holds on to more of the next." So my clients held onto quite a bit of that Mexican dinner to make up for the three meals they didn't eat. You need to stay on a schedule for your body's sake.

Any one of my clients who goes back to eating their old way is so disappointed in themselves and has all those same nasty feelings again. Bloated and tired with weight gain. You don't have to eat exactly like The Detox forever. I repeat, The Detox is not a nutrition program. It is a program to clean out your system and learn about your food reactions. It is a quick way to shed some inches and pounds the safe way.

Once you enter your fourth month, after The 90-Day Detox, you need to figure out your life eating plan. You still need to eat 4–5 complete meals a day. You can have more of a variety of foods, unlike The Detox. I have clients who choose to eat The Detox during the week and then eat what they want on weekends, still getting a meal in every three hours. The sample menus in Chapter 9, pages 52– 53, will give you examples of ways to eat once you have done The Detox. You have to decide for yourself how strict you want to be.

I tell clients to do a give-or-take method. If you take a piece of toast instead of oatmeal, then you have to give back that sandwich at lunch and have rice and chicken with veggies instead. If you take that glass of wine with your dinner, then you give back that dessert to avoid eating too much sugar in one meal. Understand? You need to keep balanced and keep in check what you are putting into your mouth. Come on! It's not that hard! You just did The 90-Day Detox for gosh sakes! See, I told you those emotions would come back here and there. You

have to keep those in check, also. So quit being a brat right now and get real with yourself! "Eat to live, don't live to eat."

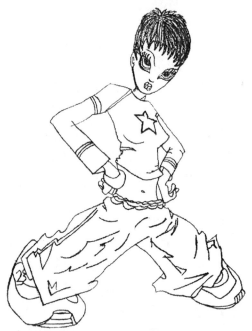

"Keep your metabolism strong... by never skipping meals!"

On the following pages, write down which good habits you need to continue and which good habits you need to develop to maintain and insure future success in your new healthy lifestyle.

19 NOBODY'S PERFECT

*"Hold yourself responsible for a higher standard
than anybody else expects of you."*
–Henry Ward Beecher

I NAMED THIS CHAPTER "NOBODY'S PERFECT" BECAUSE IT'S TRUE. THERE IS A VERY SMALL group of people who eat perfectly 24–7. What is perfect, anyway? When I used to compete in fitness competitions, I looked physically amazing, but my insides were not so healthy. I was overtrained and undernourished. Anything too extreme can cause an imbalance, which can cause trouble. I'm always amazed at how many of my clients go a little overboard with The Detox. At first they want no part of it. Once they get focused and accomplish it, I notice that they become obsessed with what they eat. They are afraid to ever eat dairy again or enjoy a sandwich or piece of pizza again. Oh, please! You have to live a little! I can't say it enough.

My Detox is only to be done to help you learn about your body physically, emotionally, and mentally. I eat The Detox way the majority of my days. I've been eating this way for 15 years now. One day a week, usually Sunday, I eat pizza or a cheeseburger or some donuts or ice cream. For me, personally, I have been on strict eating programs since I was five and started gymnastics. I learned early on how important protein was for muscle growth and performance. I enjoy eating healthy and feeling good. I also have always been a ball of energy that never sits still and I attribute most of that to my eating habits. My clients all call me a machine or crazy or weird or inspirational. I know eating my 5–6 meals a day is what keeps me going in my very active 70-hour workweeks! But I have learned in 18 years of working with all sorts of people that everyone is not the same. There is no one answer. You have to find what works for you not only physically but also mentally and emotionally.

burn, etc. Why? Their mouth is chewing gum, which signals the stomach to dump digestive enzymes, thinking the gum is coming down, which of course it doesn't. End result, built-up acid in the stomach with nothing to do but gurgle. I tell my clients to chew each bite of food 15–20 times depending on the consistency. Your food will digest easier and faster when you do this, which will keep it from storing it in your body. Chewing your food better will make you slow down when you eat.

You have to find what works for you not only physically but also mentally and emotionally.

Here are some other simple things you can do that can help you shed some inches and pounds. A real simple one, believe it or not, is to slow down and chew your food better. That's it? Yep, that's it. We have enzymes in our saliva that help break down our food while we're chewing our food. There are digestive enzymes dumping into your stomach, waiting to finish the digestion process. F.Y.I.—a lot of gum chewers have digestive problems, heart-

We are not dogs, so quit eating like one. Quit inhaling your food like someone is going to steal it! Even if you can take only 15 minutes, it's better than eating on the run in five minutes.

To help clients eat slower, I recommend they eat with chopsticks. I know these can be frustrating for some of you. Don't tell me you don't have time to fool around with these stupid things. You know, I just can't believe the disrespect some of you have for your poor little body. I'm just asking you to quit jamming your food down your throat in less than five minutes! Using chopsticks will control the amount you take in and will slow down your whole eating process. They force you to take smaller bites and give you time in between bites because you are strategically trying to pick up the next one. Come on! Try it! Your kids will love it too!

My next tip is to cut portions. You can eat the same food but just cut the portions in half and your body will start dropping some weight. I tell clients when they go out to eat to share their favorite entrée with someone or split it in half and take it home for lunch the next day. You can also order an appetizer as your main meal. Appetizers are usually the right size for one person.

As far as portions go, usually it's the size of your fist or palm of your hand. You know, they say feed a baby only the amount the size of their fist because that's the size of their stomach. Meat is usually the size of a deck of cards. A pancake is the size of a CD. A scoop of ice cream or mashed potatoes is the size of a baseball. Cheese is dice-size. Are you getting the

idea? I bet you're finding out your portions are pretty big.

Also, when you are eating out, order all your sauces on the side. Restaurants tend to drench their food. If they give you bread with your salad, eat a piece of bread with your salad, not a loaf of bread and a salad. Share a dessert instead of ordering one for yourself. Enjoy one glass of wine with dinner, not a bottle with dinner. Too much alcohol makes you not care what you are eating!

Another way to shed some pounds is to shed some water weight. One way is to drink more water. Just like the body will store more in the fat cells for every meal you miss, the body will also store more water for survival if you don't get enough. I have clients drink as close to a gallon of water a day as they can. They notice a reduction in water retention just from getting enough water.

If you take in any kind of caffeine or alcohol, you need one 8 oz. glass of water per glass of caffeine or alcohol. Why? Caffeine and alcohol are natural diuretics. They will dehydrate you. That's why a lot of people love caffeine. With it acting as a stimulant and a diuretic, they get the energy, lose some water retention, and stay regular, if you know what I mean. Most of these people don't know that too much caffeine or alcohol can have the opposite effect, forcing the body to balance itself out by purposely holding water and bloating.

Another way to lose some water weight and bloat is by dropping your complex and simple carbs. Remember earlier on I explained that carbohydrates give the muscles glycogen and any extra, unused glycogen sits on the body as extra water weight? So, if you cut out these carbohydrates which will deplete your glycogen, it will, in turn, deplete the water that goes with it. I only recommend this if you have to shed some quick pounds in less than two weeks. I tell my clients who have a party or wedding or big hoopla to go to and want to tighten down before it, that they can drop those carbohydrates for only two weeks. I also warn them that once it's over and they go back to eating they will gain at least five or more pounds back rather quickly. Most of the Hollywood stars do this trick, among others, to get ready for the big award shows they participate in so they always look awesome in those evening gowns. Most of my clients can lose anywhere from 5-

10 pounds in a week or two by using this trick. They totally understand how it's not body fat they are losing because they are so disgusted by how fast the weight comes back in less than two days after they eat normally again. But they looked awesome at their event!

Speaking of events, this is another way to motivate you to make a change with your body. Find an event, make an event, challenge a friend, a sibling, or your mate to a body makeover contest. Set a date; establish the prize, and whoever makes their goal wins! It's very motivating and healthy to challenge and compete with someone to keep you on your program.

One more very simple way to drop some pounds is to relax and get some good quality sleep! High stress and lack of sleep causes your system to hold water. Not getting good quality sleep can slow your metabolism down. I've had clients' say they went on vacation, ate whatever they wanted, and even lost some weight. I explain that they probably slept more and had better quality sleep and they were in a fun, relaxing setting with no time schedules so the body was relaxed.

What I'm trying to say in this chapter is, there are very simple ways to lose inches and weight that I'm sure a lot of you already know about and may have already tried. Just like you already know what you need to do to your eating program to change it so your body follows suit. You just have to decide what it's worth to you.

Don't worry, one day you'll have a reunion or you will be in your kid's wedding and you'll have to make a change. I just hope by then it's not too late for your health. I've had clients say, "I can't afford to be healthy, it's expensive and takes a lot of time." I always respond with, "Well, I hope you can afford to be sick. I hope you set aside enough time to be sick." It's your choice because it's your body. No one can do this for you. You're a big boy or girl now. Your momma's days of telling you to eat your vegetables are over!

YOU are responsible for what YOU put in YOUR body!

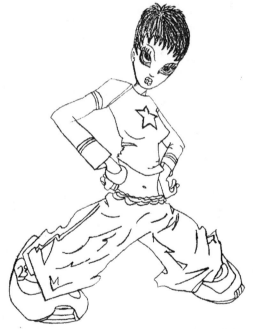

"Find balance in your relationship with food!"

20 PLAN "B"

"Failure is an event, never a person."
–William D. Brown

THIS CHAPTER IS TO HELP YOU SUCCEED. I WANT TO GIVE YOU WAYS TO BE successful. Every plan needs a Plan B. If you don't have a Plan B, you will set yourself up to fail. Why? Because as the saying goes, "shit happens." Or, as I like to say to my clients, "life happens." There is always going to be something or someone who gets in the way of your goals. It's like throwing a monkey wrench into a finely tuned machine. There will be people who will try to sabotage your new ways of life. Don't be surprised if it's your mate.

For some people, change is not a good thing. They want to keep everything status quo. It's easier this way and more comfortable. I once had a boyfriend tell me, "How about we just grow fat and old together." He said this because he hated the fact that I liked to run every night instead of sitting on the couch next to his lazy butt. I've had so-called friends go out to eat with me and say, "Are you going to eat like you always do or are you going to have fun and act normal for once?"

It's not easy making a change. Not only do you have to deal with your own issues and weaknesses, you have to deal with everyone else and their comments. I've had people say I need counseling for eating disorders just because I refused dessert at dinner. I didn't realize being focused called for counseling.

What I have learned to do is realize that these people are uncomfortable around me because their weaknesses come out. It's like the recovered alcoholic going to a party with his friends. They feel uncomfortable drinking around him. Well, food is the same way. I have never said to anyone I'm eating dinner with, "Wow, your butt really doesn't need that piece of cake you're having for dessert!" Yet everyone else has always felt the need to point out how strict I eat. This, too, will happen to you. They will say, "Oh come on, how bad is one bite going to hurt you! Try this cake!"

Do not let them make you lose your focus! Just like if this were drugs or alcohol, you may find it's in your best interest to disassociate with certain people who do not support your new goal. Otherwise, you are just going to make it that much harder on yourself. If you can't stay away from them because you happen to be married to them, then every time they try to sabotage you just say, "I could really use your support right now." Here are some other ways to help you succeed on your journey to a healthier body.

- Get out of your rut, change your routine. Take up a dance class, yoga, find a healthy restaurant, go for walks, or find a hobby.

- Find a support group or person to coach you through. Give them a cue phrase they can say to you that snaps you out of it when you go into a weak moment.

- Find someone you admire or look up to and "mirror them" or "channel them" through you. What would _____ do right now if they were in this situation.

- Pretend you are a loved one. What would you tell them right now if they were in your situation? What advice would you give them to get them through the tough spot?

You have always had all the answers. You just have to apply them. Today is that day, my friend!

The other horrible excuse I always hear is, "I have no time." My answer to that, "You don't make the time. Your time is your time. Think of a major incident in your life that you couldn't control. A death in the family, the birth of your child, an illness that took you down for a couple of days, and notice how your world kept moving. Everything survived that incident. So, when you say I don't have time because of my schedule, you are saying you do not respect yourself, you are not important to your loved ones, and, basically, you don't deserve to be healthy. So is that what you're telling me? Understand it is not easy to make a change. But realize that if it feels uncomfortable and awkward, you're probably on the right track. It's always easy to fall back into the old ways and you probably will at least a couple of times.

You need to ask yourself, what will truly make you happy?

Don't worry, this change will build personality and help you learn so much about yourself. You are ready for this! You need to envision it! If it were so damn easy, I wouldn't be sitting here on my Saturday night writing this book! We would all look amazing and be so healthy!

You need to ask yourself, what will truly make you happy? What core belief do you have deep inside that is stopping you from making your goals? Take each day as if it were your last. Focus on your goals for that day and only that day. Forgive yourself if you fail. Write down the reason you failed and put it on the fridge. Look at it in the morning and commit to not doing the same thing today. Challenge the negative little devil on your shoulder who's telling you you'll fail. Face your craving head on and talk yourself through it. If you must give in, write down what you ate and the reason why. Again, put it on the fridge and don't do the same thing tomorrow. Have fun with this. Pray to a higher power if you have to. You are building new character traits, but those old ones will always want to surface when you have a weak moment.

Notice how I said WHEN you have a weak moment. That's because life will always throw you a curve ball. DEAL WITH IT! Every time you relapse, write it down and write why you did it and put it on the fridge for the next morning. Every night, write in big letters what you did RIGHT on that day and put it next to your bed or on your bathroom mirror so you can read it when you wake up. This will help motivate you with positive affirmations that you are accomplishing your goal. The majority of people who start with excuses as to why they can't do something are usually the people who fail at the majority of the things they try. I have always lived by the phrase, "Those who say it can't be done need to move out of the way of those already doing it." Which person do you want to be?

Believe It
Be It
Become It

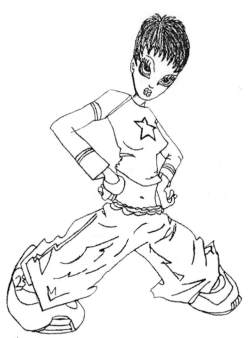

"Your body will always resemble the eating plan you stick to!"

21 HONORING THE NEW YOU

"Mastering others is strength;
mastering yourself is true power."
—Unknown

Completing Your Transformation

CHANGING YOUR EATING HABITS ALSO MEANS CHANGING YOUR LIFESTYLE. NOT ONLY will your body go through major changes physically, mentally, and emotionally but your world and the people in it will also be highly affected. Anytime you make a change and go through a change in your life, a lot of other things need to make a shift also to help that change take place. Not only do they help the change take place, but they also make sure the change becomes part of your lifestyle.

Every single one of my clients who has lost weight has gone through a rough transitional period to get there. Some have even regressed back to old ways because the changes their body made were too fast for them to mentally and emotionally handle. I had one female client, who always regressed back every time she got down to a size 8, from a size 14. After the third time around, I finally confronted her about it. She explained to me, as she broke down in tears, that she didn't know how to mentally and emotionally deal with men being attracted to her in public. If a man looked at her, or God forbid, whistled at her, because he thought she was attractive, she had an anxiety attack. She then told me, in the midst of her tears, that men don't whistle at heavy girls. So her weight was her protection, kind of like wearing armor. The reason I'm sharing this story with you is because the majority of my clients who go through any kind of weight loss go through a mental and emotional transition also. If they can't get through that and figure out what you need in your life to help you make your transition go as smoothly as possible.

Having supportive people in a supportive environment is one need all of my clients agreed was the most important. Even my 76-year-old grandma, who, by the way, lost 26 inches and dropped a couple of dress sizes on my Detox, said

You need to search deep inside your heart and soul and figure out what you need in your life...

transition and enjoy and honor their new outer appearance, they tend to regress back to old eating habits for comfort and because it's easier.

Food can be like any other addiction, very hard to break. Just like smoking, alcohol, or other drugs, you have to not only stop the use, but also make changes to your mind, your emotions, and, especially, your lifestyle. You have to change your habits, the way you do certain things, your environment, and, possibly, even the people around you. You need to search deep inside your heart and soul

she had to tell one of her friends from her church group not to bring baked goods to her anymore because she wasn't eating those types of foods as much. Her friend said, jokingly, "Why are you starving yourself, what's a bite of brownie going to hurt?" My grandma told me she did what I recommended and told her friend, "I could really use your support as my close friend right now. I have enough temptation and criticism from the rest of the world." Her friend apologized and became her biggest supporter!

I have helped my female clients find

their sexy, feminine side after losing all their inches. Instead of using baggy clothes to hide their figure, I show them how to accentuate the good in their now fit figure. I have told male and female clients to donate their clothing as they are dropping inches. That way, you need to buy new clothes and you can't go back to the old sizes. Once a client reaches their goal, I help some of them to, so-called, reinvent themselves. With their new, fit body they will wear more colors, and way different styles then ever before. Most of them go for a whole new hairstyle and the men will shave off or grow facial hair. Have fun with this process! Making these changes is part of the transitional period that helps you keep moving forward and never want to go back to your old ways again. It's saying, "Hello, world! Welcome to my new, fit body!" On top of that, you are also showing the world your true self on the inside. No more insecurities, no more hiding behind baggy clothing. You are a shining star, now be as bright as you can be!

I have taught males and females how to walk and stand and move around in their new, fit body. Please work on your posture and maybe even take a ballroom dancing class to learn how to properly stand. You can look like you have lost weight just by standing and sitting properly and not "dumping into your body." I'm sure you have all seen yourself in a picture where you are slouched over and it makes you look huge, no matter how fit you are. I always tell people to never allow your arms to rest at the sides of your body when taking a picture because it flattens your shape. So, even if you have a toned arm, it will look awful if you don't pull it away from your body. It's amazing the habits you make because of feeling insecure or unsure of yourself.

When I helped my dad lose almost 100 pounds, I had to show him how to walk and stand, and I even referred him to a chiropractor. The major weight loss on his frame caused a lot of shifting to go on in his spine and hips. Did you know that for every one pound of body fat your body holds, it puts an extra three pounds of pressure on your low back, hips, knees, ankles, and feet! So how many extra "ones" do you have? Now multiply that times three.

When my dad lost his first 50 pounds, the lower half of his body stopped aching and he moved more fluently. I took him to the pet store and had him carry a 50-pound bag of dog food around the perimeter of the store. All the pains in the lower half of his body came back, and he couldn't believe that was what he used to carry around all day. My dad also had a habit of folding his arms over his big belly when he stood in public. Once his belly was gone, he had no armrest and found that he didn't know how to just stand without feeling self-conscious about people looking at his stomach area. You need to walk with a purpose! You need to command attention in public with your stance. Show everyone you are somebody and you are proud of it! You are an important person in this world and don't you forget it!

I would have to say with all of my clients in my 20 years of helping them change their lives, the new transition and honoring their more fit outer self is actually way harder to deal with than all the work it takes to get there.

Eating right and exercising, that's the easy part. As I tell my clients, "How are you going to feel about the unveiling of this new, fit body?" Let me ask you the same question. How are YOU going to feel about unveiling YOUR new, fit body?

Are you prepared to honor yourself? Are you prepared to make the changes needed to support and nurture the needs of this new, fit body? Are you prepared to LIVE what your body is showing on the outside and not fall completely back into old habits and unhealthy ways? Don't get me wrong, we're all human; you're going to have your days where you want to eat the damn cake! And I want you to enjoy it!

Nutrition is not rocket science. I don't like diets. It is not good to completely cut out foods from your nutrition program, FOREVER! My Detox helps you learn, what foods you react to good and bad. Otherwise, losing inches is not complicated. You just choose to make it that way by adding emotions into the mix. I have had several clients say to me, "I know what to do when it comes to eating right. I just don't want to do it." And that, my friends, about sums it up! It's like we regress back to childhood when we wouldn't eat our green veggies! Those damn emotions!!

I know you will control your emotions and you will honor your new, fit body. In fact, your soul feels so good and healthy, now that you have released the athlete within you, that you will make all the changes and take care of all the needs of your new, fit body and never, ever look back into your old ways again!!

**If you don't have a goal,
You don't have a plan.
If you don't have a plan,
You don't have a direction.
If you don't have a direction,
You're standing still!**

Recap Tips

1. Eat a "complete meal," protein, complex carb, fibrous carb, good fat. Never go no carb!!!

2. Eat something every three hours to avoid having your metabolism slow down.

3. Prepare your meals in bulk ahead of time. Being unprepared means missing meals.

4. Every time you miss a meal, your body holds on to more of the next one because it thinks you're starving yourself.

5. Watch your portions. Order an appetizer for your meal, share an entrée with someone, or just take half home for your next meal.

6. Shop in the outer perimeter of the grocery store, all the junk is in the middle.

7. Use real herbs, onions, peppers, mushrooms, and tomatoes, instead of jarred, to flavor food.

8. Use low-fat, not fat-free. Fat-free foods have things in them to help the flavor and the body doesn't always recognize those.

9. Eat healthy during your week, and have a cheat day on Saturday. Eat whatever, all day, for all five meals but still keep your portions normal. This speeds up your metabolism and helps keep you sane!!

10. If you want a cheat during the week, go out to have it and be done with it. Don't buy a whole carton of ice cream, just go out for ice cream. If you have to buy large bags of chips for kids, place the right portion in individual bags when you get home and throw the big bag away.

Last but not least:

Stop making nutrition so damn complicated!!!

**You know what to do,
NOW DO IT!**

On the following pages, write down ways of honoring yourself and what things you are going to do for yourself to put yourself first and make sure you value your new, healthy lifestyle.

ACKNOWLEDGMENTS

I WOULD LIKE TO THANK MOST MY MOM AND DAD. WITHOUT THEIR HELP AND support, this book never would have been written. They sold their home of 30 years, in Illinois, to move out to Arizona to be a part of my busy world. They've helped me keep my business organized and running smoothly, along with helping me with the technical support of doing all of my computer work, which is hard for me to get to when I see over 100 appointments per week. They are amazing people and I can never tell them enough how much they are needed in my world.

I would also like to give special thanks to all of my clients, for believing in me and pushing me to get my valuable knowledge down on paper. Throughout the years, you have all been an inspiration to me.

And last but not least, I would like to thank my talented team of professionals who made this book look awesome! Tom Bird, consultant/advisor; Paul McCarthy, renowned New York editor; Jamie Saloff, awesome formatter; Julie Nelson, creative cover artist; Sharon Garner, copyeditor.

Sincerely,

Angela Jordan, A.K.A., AJ

CPSIA information can be obtained
at www.ICGtesting.com
Printed in the USA
FSOW01n0748290914
3158FS